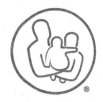

American Academy® of Husband-Coached Childbirth

Robert A. Bradley, MD
(1917 - 1998)
Co-Founder

The Bradley Method®

Dear Parents-to-be:

WELCOME. We are thrilled you have chosen to take a BRADLEY METHOD® class[...] [...]ourselves have taken Bradley® classes and are enthusiastic about the results. These classes are de[...] [...]spire you to learn, grow and become skilled in nature's birth process. Quality education is a pathway to that experience. Having a healthy baby & mother is our goal.

PROFESSIONAL TEACHERS. Bradley® teachers are professionals, having extensive training along with continuing education requirements each year. They teach because they have a desire to share with you life skills they themselves have learned through experience or observation. We are proud of our affiliated teachers for their personal attention and outstanding success in training natural childbirth students. These dedicated individuals are independent educators, trained to educate couples about natural childbirth. As teachers of The Bradley Method®, they do not practice medicine.

CLASS MATERIALS. The Student Workbook you are reading is for the exclusive use of students enrolled in Bradley® classes. Every student in every Bradley® class must receive a personal copy of this workbook. You will find a lot of information in this book. At the end of class, each couple will receive a coach-card showing they have completed our preparation program. We also ask that you note the follow-up form located in this book. Please fill out this form as soon as possible after birth and mail it back to the Academy. Your personal comments are also appreciated. We tabulate these statistics in our computer, in the hope that someday we will impress some people who do not believe in natural childbirth. Others may benefit from your sharing with us, so please take the time to return your form. Thank you. Your instructor is required to send in birth-logs on all students.

SMALL CLASSES. You have probably noticed that Bradley® classes are small and personal. This is because we have found classes of 3 to 8 couples make an ideal learning environment. When classes get too large, teachers should split them, or refer students to other affiliated teachers, locally. This way you get lots of personal attention. These classes contain 12 units of instruction as outlined in this book. The standard series has twelve weekly classes. Statistics show that 12 weeks of preparation result in more unmedicated births!

INFORMED CONSENT. Bradley® classes teach you about normality, not medicine. We also teach consumerism and encourage you to have open communications with your medical team so that you can have the best and safest birth possible. General information given in class cannot be considered the basis for giving informed consent. All information in this course is for educational purposes only! Any "Medical Advice" should be elicited from your medical professional(s). Information for informed consent must be specific to the individual mother or baby, her particular physical situation or problem and, therefore, must be given at the time the situation occurs. Information given in class can be helpful as background and will enable the couple to better communicate with their doctor about contemplated treatments. However, in order to give true informed consent for medical procedures, the couple must obtain information from many sources in advance: books, library, classes, doctor, midwife, hospital and directly from their practitioner at the time the treatment is being considered.

HELPING OTHERS. Many couples are so grateful for the classes, they write to us and ask what they can do to help others experience a natural birth. Here are some ideas: return your follow-up form soon, tell others about your experience, refer pregnant friends to your local Bradley® teachers, get a International Directory of teachers at www.bradleybirth.com, so you can refer friends across the country, take brochures where pregnant women go (maternity shops and doctors' offices), send Certificates of Appreciation to the people who helped you, tell your teacher so she can send Bradley® thank-you notes, and make sure your community has books on The Bradley Method® in the book stores and libraries.

BECOME A TEACHER. Consider becoming a teacher, yourself. There is a great need for Bradley® teachers. We need more teachers in all areas. Some people go through life looking for a way to help other people; teaching just one couple to have a beautiful birth can help make this a better world.

TAKE RESPONSIBILITY. We hope that your birth experience will be the most joyful event in your lives. In order to prepare for this, you must do your part. Your instructor will give you some information, but you must make your own decisions. We hope you will get more out of these classes than you put in. The ultimate decisions and responsibilities are yours and cannot be delegated to others. Many issues are still controversial and unresolved. Every intervention has potential risks, as well as possible benefits. You, as parents, will live the rest of your lives with the choices you make now; you alone will raise your child ... not your teacher, doctor, midwife, birth center or hospital. Choose wisely.

THE CHALLENGE. We, at the Academy, challenge you to take your responsibility as parents seriously. We really believe in NATURE and the natural way. Learn as much as you can from as many different sources as possible. Remember, pregnancy is normal, not an illness. The natural process has worked for countless generations. Help it work for you. Good luck and remember, there is so much to learn, so little time. Make the most of this time.

Your baby is counting on you!

Marjie Hathaway

Sincerely,

*HW: Fears pkt
nutrition / exercises
read lesson 4 binder
bring pillows
practice massage
Study help topic*

1/15/12

TABLE OF CONTENTS

©2010 AAHCC

WAYS OF HANDLING PAIN

Check off ways you have handled pain in the past:

Discuss in class which ways would be helpful in labor. Those items in *bold* may help you avoid unnecessary pain.

❏ Close Eyes	❏ *Silence	❏ *Image of Special Place
❏ *Sleep*	❏ *Music	❏ *Wipe Forehead
❏ Cry	❏ *Journal / Write Down Feelings	❏ *Praise
❏ *X* Drugs	❏ *Abdominal Breathing*	❏ *Call Doctor
❏ *Hot Water Bottle	❏ *Analyze	❏ *Brush Hair
❏ Bath	❏ *Distraction	❏ Candles
❏ *Massage	❏ *Eat*	❏ *Foot Rub
❏ *Ice	❏ *Drink Water*	❏ *Ice Chips
❏ Scream	❏ Grit Your Teeth	❏ Let Go
❏ *Ignore	❏ *Go to the Bathroom - Urinate*	❏ Pet(s)
❏ Think About Pain	❏ *Walk it Off*	❏ Vocalize
❏ *Put Pressure on It*	❏ *Dark / Light	❏ _____
❏ *Privacy	❏ *Change Position*	❏ _____
❏ *Company	❏ *Not Lying on Your Back*	❏ _____
❏ *Sympathy	❏ *Understanding / Education*	❏ _____
❏ *Seek Comfort	❏ *Back Rub	❏ _____
❏ *Support	❏ *Relax*	❏ _____
❏ Deal with It	❏ Dress Comfortably	❏ _____
❏ Accept It	❏ *Shower	❏ _____

The American Academy of Pediatrics, Committee on Drugs has stated: "No drug or chemical - whether prescription, over-the-counter or food additive - can be regarded as having been proven to be entirely free of potential harm to the fetus." Pediatrics. Vol. 51 No. 2. "Development of the Blood-Brain Barrier. The cerebral capillaries are much more permeable at birth than in adulthood, and the blood-brain barrier develops during the early years of life." *Review of Medical Physiology*, 16th edition, 1993.

Class 1 Class 2 Class 3 Class 4 Class 5 Class 6 Class 7 Class 8 Class 9 Class 10 Class 11 Class 12

THE _____ FAMILY STUDENT WORKBOOK

Family Portrait
(during pregnancy)

Estimated Due Date:

/   /

Today's Date:

/   /

(Harvard public health study shows an average of 41 1/7 weeks gestation.)

Class 1 Class 2 Class 3 Class 4 Class 5 Class 6 Class 7 Class 8 Class 9 Class 10 Class 11 Class 12

Pre-Birth Bonding

It is our hope that filling out this workbook will help you to feel closer to your baby both during pregnancy and after it is born. Babies function before birth. Hearing starts around 24 weeks, so read, talk, sing, & play music to your baby during pregnancy. Write a letter to your baby expressing your feelings during this time of your life.

We are looking forward to: *(seeing, touching, loving, holding you, etc.)*

We are excited about: *(being parents, etc.)*

We are concerned about: *(finances, parenting, etc.)*

We are preparing for your birth by:

We think our baby is going to be a: ❑ Boy, ❑ Girl, ❑ Twins

"Ultrasound examinations performed solely to satisfy the family's desire to know the fetal sex, view the fetus, or to obtain a picture of the fetus should be discouraged." National Institutes of Health Consensus Development Conference Statement, Volume 5, Number 1.

Class 1 · Class 2 · Class 3 · Class 4 · Class 5 · Class 6 · Class 7 · Class 8 · Class 9 · Class 10 · Class 11 · Class 12

Pregnancy Goals

The following are statements often made about childbirth. Mark them True or False. Then, fill in the title line above.

TRUE *FALSE*

1. A natural, totally unmedicated childbirth is something few women can accomplish, especially those having their first baby.

2. Husbands always faint in the delivery room. It is better for a husband to stay out.

3. It is all right if your nutrition is not as good as it should be when you're pregnant because the baby can take what it needs from the mother.

4. The placenta acts as a barrier, so that drugs and other potentially harmful things are unable to reach the baby.

5. Since childbirth is a natural function, women don't need to go to classes, but can rely on their instincts to get them through it.

6. The key to The Bradley Method® of natural birth is to use the proper designated breathing pattern for each stage of labor.

7. Disassociation and distraction are the only ways to control pain in childbirth.

8. Babies are blind at birth.

9. Bottle feeding is just as good as breastfeeding

10. What you don't know can't hurt you.

11. Having a baby in the best hospital insures that you won't be responsible if anything goes wrong.

12. Having gone through The Bradley Method® classes does you no good if you end up with a cesarean section.

We want you to have the safest and most rewarding birth experience possible. The primary goal is a healthy mother, baby, & family. For that reason, we endorse and teach the following:

1. Natural Childbirth - *Over 86% of Bradley® moms having vaginal births do so without medication.*

2. Active participation of the husband as coach.

3. Excellent nutrition, the foundation of a healthy pregnancy & baby.

4. Avoidance of drugs during pregnancy, birth, and breastfeeding - unless absolutely necessary. *No drug has been proven safe for an unborn baby.*

5. Training: "Early-Pregnancy" classes followed by weekly classes starting in the 5th to 6th month, continuing until birth.

6. Relaxation and NATURAL breathing - *Can be effective pain management techniques with training according to the National Institutes of Health.*

7. "Tuning-in" to your own body and trusting the natural process.

8. Immediate and continuous contact with your new baby.

9. Breastfeeding, beginning at birth, provides immunities & nutrition.

10. Consumerism and positive communications.

11. Parents taking responsibility for the safety of the birth place, procedures, attendants, and emergency back-up.

12. Preparation for unexpected situations such as emergency childbirth and cesarean section.

Educated parents have the responsibility to make these choices themselves and to hire the personnel who will support their choices. This takes considerable effort and sometimes requires changing your situation or traveling great distances to seek the safest possible birth.

Your local independent Bradley Method® instructor is a professional person or couple trained to educate couples about natural childbirth. These instructors have gone through intensive training by the American Academy of Husband-Coached Childbirth® and are required to re-affiliate each year in order to continue teaching The Bradley Method®. *Currently Affiliated Instructors are listed on:* www.bradleybirth.com.

STAYING HEALTHY AND LOW RISK

The first responsibility of becoming a mother is to stay healthy and low risk. Pregnancy is generally a very healthy time of life, and birth is an inherently safe process. Occasionally there are risk factors that are out of your control such as genetic problems, disease or injury. These things are rare, but may put you into a high risk category that would require your working even closer with your medical team and, perhaps, choosing some interventions necessary for the health of the mother and baby. Low risk mothers have more choices.

The following is an outline of 5 suggestions on what you can do to stay healthy and low risk. They may help you to avoid complications. If a complication does occur, starting with a healthy mother and baby will affect the outcome in a positive way. Discuss the details of these suggestions.

1. Nutrition:
    A. Good nutrition helps avoid toxemia, premature rupture of membranes (PROM) & hypovolemia.
    B. Well-balanced diet.
    C. 80-100 grams of protein daily.
    D. Salt to taste and water to thirst.

2. Exercise:
    A. Regular physical exercise for stamina.
    B. Pregnancy exercises for preparation for birth.

3. Taking Responsibility:
    A. Being informed.
    B. Avoiding substances that could be harmful.
    C. Avoiding procedures unless necessary.

4. Education:
    A. Books i.e. *Husband-Coached Childbirth, Children at Birth, Natural Childbirth The Bradley® Way, Assistant Coach's Manual,* etc.
    B. Friends & family.
    C. Health Care Provider.
    D. Bradley® classes.
    E. Visit Student Center on: www.bradleybirth.com

5. Relaxation:
    A. Practicing techniques daily.
    B. Avoiding and alleviating stress.
    C. Getting plenty of rest.

©2010 AAHCC

PARENTAL DECISIONS AND NEONATAL HEALTH

by Joseph William Hazell, M.P.H.

There is a large body of established knowledge and belief upon which nearly all physicians agree, but there are also important areas where they disagree. In these areas of disagreement, decisions are shifted to the patient who makes them (often unknowingly) by his choice of a physician. This is quite as true of obstetrics as of any medical field.

The kind of pregnancy, labor and delivery our children experience has a profound and lifelong effect on their health, particularly their mental and emotional health. As things stand today, a number of important decisions about a particular childbirth are made by the parents at the time they choose their physicians.

While it is the mother who cannot avoid ultimate responsibility for choosing how her child will be born, her decisions are influenced by many experiences, a most important one being the concern of the father of her child. As fathers-to-be, we inevitably share in this decision process, even if by default, and thus profoundly affect the health of our children.

A significant health risk that can be improved by the choice of a physician is that of minimal brain damage. By this is meant a host of mental and behavioral disabilities that still leave a child within normal ranges. Lowered intelligence, speech and reading difficulties, shortened attention span, awkward physical coordination and hyperactivity have all been associated with conditions of stress imposed by drug use and position during labor.

The still common use of drugs, instead of relaxation techniques as the method of choice for pain relief during labor, remains a major form of drug abuse in this country. Even cigarette smoking and aspirin offer measurable risks during pregnancy and evidence is increasing that amounts of drugs sufficient to provide pain relief during labor are also enough to substantially stress the baby. Nevertheless, some physicians who will insist on avoiding certain drugs and dosages when a premature baby is expected will either offer or allow an uninformed mother to choose these same drugs and dosages when a baby is expected to be out of risk of actual death. Death is a visible failure. Minimal brain damage is often invisible. It's your child and it is you who choose the policy on drug use during his or her birth when you choose your physician.

Though it has long been known that an upright position during second stage is often more comfortable, it is only in recent years that there has been clear evidence that lying on the back or leaning back during any part of labor can sometimes put severe stress on the oxygen supply to the baby. What can happen, without the mother or physician even being aware of it, is pressure of the heavy uterus on the inferior vena cava, ultimately reducing blood flow to the placenta. This loss of oxygen, or partial asphyxia, especially during the exertions of labor, results in injury to brain cells and is one of the causes of minimal brain damage. An upright delivery avoids this pressure problem as well as often feeling much more comfortable. It's your child, and when you choose a physician you also choose a policy on how position will affect your child's oxygen supply during labor.

Another important health risk that can be improved by choice of a physician is that of prematurity. A baby born before it is mature enough, or big enough to survive easily, can either die or survive with whatever effects may remain from the fight for survival. Two common but avoidable procedures that substantially increase the likelihood of prematurity or of dangerously low birth weight are dieting during pregnancy and elective induction.

It used to be a common belief, and still is among some physicians, that weight gain beyond various arbitrary limits tended to produce toxemia of pregnancy which, in turn, increases the risk of prematurity and stillbirth. Now, the National Research Council Committee on Maternal Nutrition observes that there is no evidence for that view and points out that, quite the contrary, strict weight control, itself, contributes to low birth weight and stillbirth. It is far more important to have a full range of sound nutrition than to limit natural weight gain. It's your child, and you are influencing its birth weight when you choose a physician.

There was a time when elective induction was touted as a great convenience because one could go into labor by appointment and not keep obstetricians up at night. It soon appeared that even with good physical examinations and counting from the last missed period, there were too many premature inductions. It turned out, too, that drug-induced labor sometimes coincided with natural labor and the combination produced extended contractions which interfered seriously with blood circulation. Today, there appears to be a revival of elective induction because of the "pill." A woman who stops taking the pill in order to get pregnant may not start to have periods or to ovulate regularly and immediately. Unfortunately, some physicians who assume that conception occurs soon after the pill is stopped convince themselves that nine months later they have an overdue baby who should be induced. If one doesn't know when conception occurred, a little patience may be better than premature forced induction of labor. It's your child, and when you choose a physician you also help set the risk of premature induction.

We and our children live our lives with the consequences of these decisions. Let us not choose blindly.

EXERCISE

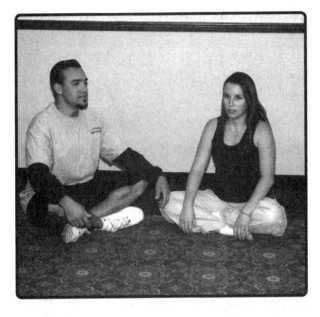

Core temperature: temperature in the innermost part of the body, normal is around 98.6 degrees Fahrenheit.

Kegel: name for the pelvic floor muscle (pubococcygeous), or exercises to strengthen it. (discovered by Dr. Arnold Kegel)

Pelvic floor: supportive muscle surrounding the urethra, vagina and rectum, extends from symphysis pubis in front to coccyx in back.

Pelvis: basin-like ring of bone at the bottom of the mother's spine through which the baby must pass to be born.

Pubic bone: symphysis pubis, is the front portion of the pelvis.

Pubococcygeous muscle: also called the PC muscle and the pelvic floor muscle. Supports the abdominal organs and uterus. (see Kegel)

Rectum: portion of large intestine connected to the anus.

Stamina: resistance to fatigue; endurance; staying power.

Urethra: tube which carries urine from bladder to exterior of body.

Uterus: "baby box", hollow muscular organ in which the baby grows and is nourished, also called the womb.

Giving birth to a baby is a physically active event, involving many special muscles and a lot of hard work. Other animals, including dolphins, prepare for birth by exercising during pregnancy. This natural childbirth preparation program stresses the importance of regular physical exercise, plus special pregnancy exercises. Your physical condition when you give birth will make a difference.

Most activities can be continued safely during pregnancy. If it causes pain, don't do it and consult with your medical team. Be careful and use common sense; avoid lying on your back; avoid excessive pressure on the Kegel muscle (i.e. jogging or bouncing); avoid putting too much stress on your body (keep your pulse and core temperature in a normal range); and check with your health care birth team if you have any questions or concerns.

TENSE/RELAX TECHNIQUE

We will begin this series of relaxation techniques with a simple example of tension vs. relaxation. Coach, get your partner in the side relaxation position and help her to adjust the pillows comfortably. Start by having her tense her right foot. Have her pull her toes up toward her head and tense all the way up her leg. Coach, feel that tension. Say aloud, "This is tension. This is what it feels like. This is what we will avoid in labor." Now, tell her to relax, and massage all the tension out of that leg. As you massage away the tension, say aloud, "This is relaxation. This is good. This is what we will use in labor." Next have her tense and then relax her left leg. Continue by progressively tensing then relaxing each muscle group in her body. Don't forget her shoulders, neck, and face. This technique can be used during contractions in labor and will prepare you for the next technique.

GENERAL ASSIGNMENTS

☐ Relaxation: 10 min. 2X a day.

☐ Walking: 5 min. 1X a day.

☐ Tailor Sitting: Often.

☐ Squat: Often.

☐ Butterfly: (3) 1X a day.

☐ Pelvic Rock: (10) 4X+20 at bedtime.

☐ Kegel: 50X a day.

☐ Complete Pink Nutrition Worksheet.

☐ *Husband-Coached Childbirth*: Get this book!

☐ *Go to Student Center on:* www.bradleybirth.com .

Class 1 | Class 2 | Class 3 | Class 4 | Class 5 | Class 6 | Class 7 | Class 8 | Class 9 | Class 10 | Class 11 | Class 12

Class 1
Class 2
Class 3
Class 4
Class 5
Class 6
Class 7
Class 8
Class 9
Class 10
Class 11
Class 12

EXERCISE DURING PREGNANCY

Pregnant women need to be aware of their bodies. "Tuning-in" to and paying attention to your bodily needs are things only you can do. These exercises have been done by thousands of pregnant women who have found them to be a great help. Women who are experiencing any complications during pregnancy, have any back, neck or knee injuries, or experience any discomfort while doing these exercises should use caution and check with their health care providers before beginning this or any exercise program.* They all should be done slowly and with control. The number you do each day will depend on your condition. In any case, start slowly and gradually increase the number you do each day. If you have any questions about these exercises or have a special medical problem, please consult with your birth team.

Regular Physical Exercise

It is important to get some kind of exercise every day so that you will have the stamina it takes to labor and give birth. This can be done any number of ways. *Be careful of balance, avoid risk of abdominal trauma, avoid becoming dehydrated and/or exhausted, and avoid anything that hurts.*

1. Many women choose to continue doing some sport or form of exercise that they are used to doing regularly (i.e. bicycling, hiking, going to exercise classes, etc.). You may need to modify the intensity of exercise according to maternal symptoms.

2. Pregnant women often like to swim because it almost makes them feel like they are not pregnant. It reduces the pressure on legs and pelvis. The water pressure also makes swollen feet and ankles feel better.

3. Walking is an excellent way of getting exercise and almost every one can do it. By taking a couple of long, reflective walks each day you can get in your daily exercise while also reducing stress, aiding your digestion, and naturally and rhythmically helping to align your spine.

Pregnancy Exercises

These exercises taught in Bradley® classes are designed specifically to tone and condition the muscles you will use to give birth. These exercises also aid in minimizing many common pregnancy discomforts.

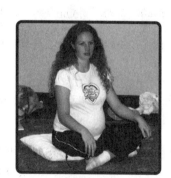

1. TAILOR SITTING

This is a healthy, natural position, although uncommon in our society. This posture encourages the uterus to move forward, increasing circulation and stretching the inner thighs.

Sit on the floor or firm pillow with your legs crossed. Remember good posture. Variation is good, lean forward or backward against something, stretch your legs occasionally. Change position often.

Start with a short period of time. Gradually make tailor sitting a way of life. It can be fun.

HOW THE COACH CAN HELP: Join in this exercise on the floor. Encourage her to tailor sit whenever possible. Explain to friends and relatives how important this is and have them sit on the floor too. Remind her to move around often.

* Reflects recommendations from The American College of Obstetricians and Gynecologists (ACOG Technical Bulletin #189).

2. SQUATTING

Squatting is a common position used in many cultures. It can be especially beneficial for giving birth. You will probably be trying to imitate this position for the birth, even if you are on a delivery table or birthing bed. Squatting gets the body in the natural alignment to put pressure on the uterus, to prevent arching of the back (which interferes with pushing), to shorten the birth canal, and to increase the outlet of the pelvis by more than 10%. It generally shortens second stage. This exercise also helps to prepare the leg muscles. It is important for the preparation of the perineum.

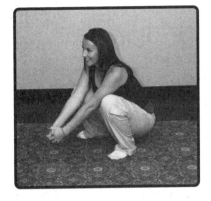

Start by standing straight, with legs comfortably apart. Next, bend knees slightly & tuck hips under (to relieve pressure on the lower back). Then, bend forward (to help keep uterus forward) and squat, keeping heels on the floor. When coming up, do so tail-first halfway, then place hands on legs (to help support lower back) as you come up the rest of the way. Your instructor will show you how to do this exercise with your coach. Some women need to practice for a while before they can get their heels on the floor. If necessary, hang on to something supportive or wear low heels.

As you become more comfortable with this exercise, do it more frequently throughout the day. Avoid bending over; squat instead.

HOW THE COACH CAN HELP: Remind her to squat every time she goes down to pick up light things. If she has trouble, squat holding on to each other as shown in class.

3. PELVIC ROCKING

This exercise probably produces more benefits than any other pregnancy exercise. It tones and conditions the muscles of the lower back and abdominal muscles; it relieves pressure (on lower back, major blood vessels, ureters, and bladder); it increases circulation, relieves general tension, and often improves digestion. When done properly, this exercise helps the baby come forward, relieving pressure.

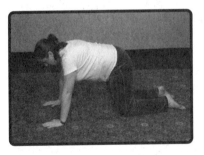

In hands and knees position (hands and knees should form a box), relax lower back, allowing pelvis to tilt forward (comfortably), then level and tuck hips under (do slowly and rhythmically with control). This exercise moves the lower part of the body only.

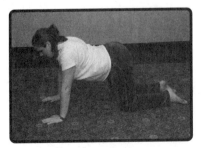

Do for brief and frequent periods throughout the day, before relaxation practices, and at bed time.

HOW THE COACH CAN HELP: Place your hand (using light pressure) on her lower back to give her an area she can concentrate on, if necessary. Remind her to do this exercise before going to bed, even if she is tired; she and the baby may sleep more comfortably.

Class 1
Class 2
Class 3
Class 4
Class 5
Class 6
Class 7
Class 8
Class 9
Class 10
Class 11
Class 12

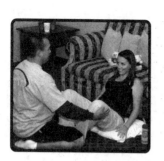

4. BUTTERFLY

This exercise tones and conditions abductor muscles and enables you to pull your legs back more comfortably in the second stage of labor. It also helps reduce shaking of legs after the birth and unnecessary pain.

The pregnant woman sits on floor leaning back against a wall or furniture with knees up and feet together, flat on the floor. Coach places flats of hands on the outside of her knees and applies resistance while the mother tries to open her legs. Remember, this is not a contest; only apply resistance when legs are going down, not on the way up. Legs need only go down as far as comfortable.

This is a powerful exercise, so 3-10 times once a day is plenty.

HOW THE COACH CAN HELP: Your active help is needed for this one. Apply resistance only; this is not a contest. As she gets stronger, apply a little more pressure. Do not overdo this exercise: it is a powerful one.

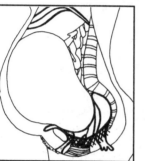

POOR TONE and SAGGING POSITIONS

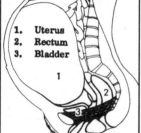

1. Uterus
2. Rectum
3. Bladder

GOOD TONE and PROPER POSITIONS

5. KEGEL/PUBOCOCCYGEUS

This exercise helps maintain proper tone in the pelvic floor or pubococcygeus muscle. Poor tone may cause: incontinence - wetting pants when coughing or sneezing; discomfort; lack of sensation during intercourse; unusual pain during birth; premature flexion of baby's head; prolonged second stage; damage to muscle; and feelings of pressure.

Tighten your Kegel muscle. It feels as if you are pulling everything in your pelvic area up. Then, relax.

Do this exercise many times a day, increasing each day.

HOW THE COACH CAN HELP: The hardest part of this exercise is remembering to do it. Please remind her often. It is also a good exercise for coaches (men have this muscle, too).

6. SIDE RELAXATION AND SLEEP POSITION

This is a safe and comfortable position for sleeping and in labor. This position helps circulation and allows the bed to support the baby's weight. It is also important during labor, to reduce stress or strain on body parts and enabling the uterus to work unencumbered.

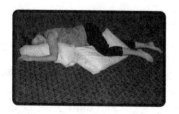

Start on your side with both knees slightly bent and the top leg forward. Your pillow should be at an angle under your head and breast. Your bottom arm may be behind you; if that's uncomfortable, bring it around over the top of your head.

Practice twice a day, once alone and once with your coach. This position may also be used for sleep.

HOW THE COACH CAN HELP: Remind her to do this exercise and practice with her once a day. Learn how she likes her back rubbed in her pregnant state. Massage tension away.

RELAXATION

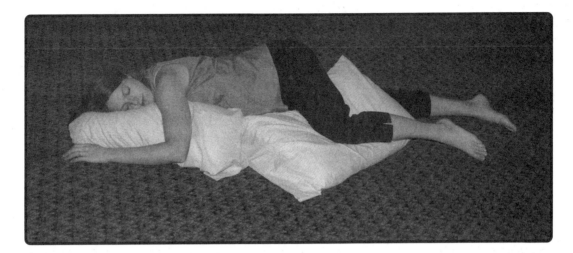

RELAXATION IS THE KEY

Relaxation is the key to The Bradley Method® during labor. It is the safest and most effective way to reduce unnecessary pain and to handle any pain you do experience.

IT TAKES PRACTICE

Relaxation is a learned response. It is something which you should practice every day. With practice, you should be able to work together so well that the mother will be able to completely relax immediately in response to the coach's voice and touch. You must work to achieve this goal.

THERE ARE THREE TYPES OF RELAXATION

Through these classes, we will deal with the three types of relaxation: physical, mental and emotional. Physical relaxation deals with the ability to relax the muscles in your body as you release tension. Mental relaxation has to do with what you are thinking about or concentrating on. Emotional relaxation has to do with how you feel about what is happening.

YOU NEED TO PRACTICE EVERY DAY

We encourage you to practice relaxation at least twice a day for up to 20 minutes each time. If necessary, the mother should practice once by herself and once with her coach.

CONCENTRATE AS YOU PRACTICE

Be sure to take this time very seriously. Mother, keep your mind active and concentrate on relaxing. Keep your eyes closed. Pretend that you are in labor, if you can. Coach, pay attention. Is she as relaxed as she can be? You must convey relaxation through your touch, through your voice, and through your actions. It may not be easy for her to concentrate and relax for very long; praise her for her efforts and recognize her progress. Remember, the better you can work together to achieve deep relaxation in practice, the better it will work in labor.

PRACTICE IN VARIOUS SITUATIONS

During your labor you will need to be relaxed, because you will be working very hard. Your mind will be quite active and you will be concentrating. You may be walking, sitting, watching TV, cleaning the house, pelvic rocking, taking a shower, bath, or lying down. So, practice relaxing at various times and in various places.

YOU'LL LEARN A SERIES OF TECHNIQUES. BE SURE TO MASTER ALL OF THEM.

Through the course of these classes, we will teach you a number of different relaxation techniques that you will need to practice. Each week we will demonstrate a technique. Practice until you feel you have really mastered a technique. If you are having difficulty with any technique, check with your instructor. Note which techniques seem to work best, but master them all, because you never know what you'll need in labor.

Class 1 | Class 2 | Class 3 | Class 4 | Class 5 | Class 6 | Class 7 | Class 8 | Class 9 | Class 10 | Class 11 | Class 12

STUDY HELPS

1. Which exercise helps the uterus to come forward and encourages good circulation while it tones and conditions your inner thighs? It also helps to prevent varicose veins.

2. Which exercise tones and conditions your perineum, helping you to avoid an episiotomy or a tear? It is also an ideal position to give birth in, as it gets the body in the natural alignment to apply downward pressure on the uterus, to prevent arching of the back (which interferes with pushing), and to shorten the birth canal. It also increases the opening of the outlet of the bony pelvis by more than 10%.

3. Which exercise tones and conditions the muscle which controls the urethra, vagina, and the rectum and is responsible for the female sexual climax? The baby must pass through this muscle during second stage. Having done this exercise regularly during pregnancy can help to avoid unnecessary damage to this muscle and unnecessary pain for the mother.

4. Which exercise tones and conditions the abductor muscles so that you will be better able to hold your legs back comfortably during second stage? Having done this exercise regularly can help to prevent the problem of sore, shaking legs that comes from muscle fatigue in second stage.

5. What exercise are you doing regularly to get the over-all strength and stamina it will take to give birth to your baby?

6. Which exercise is good for backaches and many other discomforts associated with pregnancy? It gets the uterus out of the pelvis, which makes you more comfortable and improves your circulation, as it tones and conditions the abdominal muscles.

7. Which position helps avoid the dangers of lying on your back by maintaining good circulation and is one of the most conducive to relaxation?

8. The Bradley Method® teaches that giving birth is an athletic _____. That is why we call the husbands _____.

9. The pregnancy exercises are designed to tone and condition the three B's:_____, _____ and _____.

NUTRITION

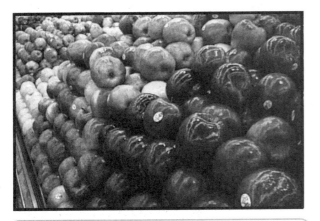

Anemia: lower than normal amount of red blood cells in the blood, sometimes called low blood count.

Balanced diet: a harmonious proportion of parts or elements in the diet. Supplying all essential and supplemental nutrients in their proper balance.

Dehydration: excessive loss of water from the body.

Deficiency: absence of something essential; shortage; deficit.

Hypovolemia: absence of normal increase, or abnormally decreased volume of circulating blood in the body.

Nutrients: essential substances which affect the metabolic and growth processes in the mother or the baby.

Pica: a craving for unusual foods during pregnancy.

Pre-eclampsia: also called toxemia; those symptoms often believed to be predictive of eclampsia; edema, proteinuria and hypertension.

Protein: organic substances essential in the diet, containing amino acids; primary substances for human life and growth.

Toxemia: also called pre-eclampsia, life-threatening disease of pregnancy leading to eclampsia (convulsions).

Good nutrition in pregnancy is important for normal development, growth, and functioning of your unborn baby. Poor nutrition can result in a premature and/or low birth weight baby with an increased risk of mental and physical problems. Proper nutrition is also important for the mother whose goal is normal reproduction, growth, energy, and health. Lack of food could cause the mother to have anemia, infections, placental malfunctions, low blood volume, difficult labor, cesarean surgery, poor healing, toxemia or pre-eclampsia, and problems with breastfeeding. Every effort should be made to attain and maintain an adequate, balanced daily intake of all the necessary nutrients throughout pregnancy.

Here are some tools and information to help you maintain a well-balanced diet during this pregnancy. Nutrition work sheets can be obtained from your Bradley® instructor. The recommendations in this section are based on information from the Brewer medical diet in the book *What Every Pregnant Woman Should Know*, USDA, and the California Department of Health. Substitutions should be made in case of allergies, dislikes, etc., but do so carefully and consider the various components of each food group.

PROGRESSIVE RELAXATION

Start by reviewing the tense/relax technique. Then imagine you are in the shower or under a gentle waterfall on a warm day in Hawaii. Feel the water as it flows over your head and down the back of your head and your face. Smell the freshness and let your body absorb the moisture as you relax your head neck and shoulders. Notice how the water cascades over your shoulders in smooth sheets and caresses your arms, elbows, wrist and each finger as it drains off your hands. Just let go of these muscles as they begin to feel the relaxing sensation of this warm water. Next feel the water run down your back and hips and down your neck, breasts, and abdomen. Feel these muscles releasing and letting go. Think about how relaxing this must be to your baby. Warm, safe, and comfortable. Now focus on the water flowing down your legs, to knees, to ankles, to feet, and toes as it washes away the tension and pressure of the day. Be sure that the pace of your speech and the tone of your voice lowers as you assist her to become more and more relaxed. This technique can be used during contractions or even between contractions in hard labor to achieve deep relaxation.

GENERAL ASSIGNMENTS

- ☐ Tailor sit: often.
- ☐ Squat: often.
- ☐ Butterfly: (5) 1X a day.
- ☐ Pelvic Rock: (20) 4X + 40 at bedtime.
- ☐ Kegel: 100X a day.
- ☐ Walk: 5 min 2X a day.
- ☐ Relax: 10 min 2X a day.
- ☐ Fill out Pink Nutrition Worksheet.
- ☐ *Husband-Coached Childbirth*
       Read chapters 1 - 2.
- ☐ Fill out *Student Workbook*; page 16.
- ☐ Go to Student Center on: www.bradleybirth.com

Class 1 | Class 2 | Class 3 | Class 4 | Class 5 | Class 6 | Class 7 | Class 8 | Class 9 | Class 10 | Class 11 | Class 12

Dr. Brewer Suggests...

ELEMENTS OF A WELL-BALANCED DIET

Each day your baby needs you to eat a well-balanced diet including all of the nutrients represented in each category. (If you are allergic to any of these foods, make substitutions carefully!)

MILK PRODUCTS - Provide protein, calcium and other essential vitamins and minerals. It is important for bones, muscle growth, muscle contraction and nerve transmission. Essential for healthy blood, eases insomnia, and helps regulate the heartbeat. Recommendation: 4 servings per day.

List your 2 favorite foods containing milk:

_____,_____

EGGS - Provide protein, vitamins and minerals, including vitamin A, the anti-infection vitamin. Added together, milk and eggs provide a protein, vitamin, mineral, and calorie foundation for the rest of the diet. Recommendation: 2 per day.

List your 2 favorite egg dishes:

_____,_____

PROTEIN - Provides amino acids which are the building blocks of the body. Important for healthy bones, teeth, muscles, brain, everything. Inadequate protein intake can lead to fatigue, swelling, and a lack of appetite. Recommendation: 2 servings per day.

List your 2 favorite protein foods:

_____,_____

GREENS - Fresh, dark green vegetables are rich in vitamins and minerals, particularly A and B complex, which are necessary to help your body use the protein in other foods. These are also high in folic acid, which is essential for good growth. Greens also play a role in the formation of red blood cells. A deficiency could lead to anemia. The darker the green, the higher the concentration of vitamins and minerals. Recommendation: 2 servings per day.

List your 2 favorite green vegetable dishes:

_____,_____

WHOLE GRAINS (breads and cereals) - These are excellent sources of carbohydrates you need to fuel your body. If you have too few carbohydrates, your body burns the protein you eat for energy, thus robbing you and your baby of the building blocks for tissue growth and repair. Carbohydrates from whole grains also are a good source of B vitamins, which are necessary for growth and the normal functioning of nerve tissue. Recommendation: 4 or more servings per day.

List your 2 favorite uses for breads and cereals:

_____,_____

CITRUS (and other high vitamin C foods) - Vitamin C is important for the body's manufacture of collagen, the substance that holds tissue together. Without adequate vitamin C, your uterus is not as strong and may not perform well in labor. Vitamin C is crucial in the body's defense system against infection and in improving iron absorption. Recommendation: 1-2 servings per day.

List your 2 favorite vitamin C foods:

_____,_____

BUTTER (fats and oils) - Fats and oils are needed to help your body absorb the fat-soluble vitamins A, D, E & K. Fats and oils also contribute to a fine-textured (stretchable) skin. They are concentrated sources of calories. The food energy or calorie need is greatly increased during pregnancy to a minimum of 2500-3000 calories per day. Recommendation: 3 servings per day.

List your 2 favorite ways to include fats/oils in your diet:

_____,_____

YELLOW AND ORANGE-COLORED FRUITS AND VEGETABLES-These foods are high in vitamin A, which is known for its role in preventing infection. During pregnancy, when the pressure of the growing uterus on the bladder is constant, extra vitamin A helps protect you against bladder and kidney infections. Recommendation: 5 servings per week.

List your 2 favorite orange or yellow foods:

_____,_____

SALT - An essential nutrient. Cutting back on salt can cause a decrease in the amount of blood circulating through your body and placenta (hypovolemia), thus reducing the supply of nutrients passing to your baby. Too little salt in the diet leads to leg cramps and fatigue. Recommendation: salt your food to taste.

List 2 sources of salt in your diet:

_____,_____

WATER (fluids) - Water accounts for 75% of your baby's total body weight at birth. It acts as a solvent and catalyst for biological reactions. Lack of water leads to dehydration, which can lead to over 20% reduction of energy output. Dehydration can also lead to headaches during pregnancy. Recommendation: drink to thirst.

List 2 sources of fluids:

_____,_____

©2010 AAHCC

Class 1 | Class 2 | Class 3 | Class 4 | Class 5 | Class 6 | Class 7 | Class 8 | Class 9 | Class 10 | Class 11 | Class 12

NUTRITION FOR YOUR NEW BABY
Breastfeeding Questionnaire

Note: The American Academy of Pediatrics policy on breastfeeding states that exclusive breastfeeding is the ideal nutrition for babies beginning as soon as possible after birth. Newborns should be nursed whenever they show signs of hunger. Pediatrics, Volume 100, Number 6, December, 1997.

Read, The Womanly Art of Breastfeeding & attend La Leche League meetings

1. Is bottle feeding or pumped milk just as good as a baby nursing directly from the breast? *no*

2. How soon after birth can a baby nurse? What is your birth team's policy? *immediately*

3. What is the name of the fluid which comes from the mother's breasts at the time of birth? Why is it important? *colostrum – antibodies, easily digestible, densely caloric, encourages meconium passage*

4. What is a normal weight loss for babies after birth? *10%*

5. When does the milk come in? *3–5 days*

6. Do babies need to be given formula until the milk comes in? *no*

7. What is engorgement? What can you do to help prevent it? If you do become engorged, what will make you more comfortable? *fill up - turn into rocks* *nursing often* *regular feedings, pump cold/warm compress*

8. How is the amount of milk you will have determined? *by need, demand*

9. How often do newborn babies, on the average, nurse? *every 2 hours – 3 hours 8-12x/day* *start of one to start of next*

10. Do babies need an occasional bottle of formula, juice, or water? *no*

11. What problems can be caused by giving an occasional bottle? *not want to breastfeed, loss of supply, nipple confusion*

12. What are the differences between breast and bottle-fed babies? *more healthy, smarter – higher IQ, smell better, different body fat, getting antibodies, less allergys*

13. Does your birth place or your back-up birth place routinely give babies a bottle while they're in the nursery? *no*
    How do you feel about this?

14. Can a woman with inverted nipples nurse her baby?

15. Can a woman with very small breasts nurse her baby? *yes*

16. Can a woman with very large breasts nurse her baby?

17. Can a woman who has twins or triplets nurse her babies?

18. Should most babies stop breastfeeding because of jaundice? *no*

Dam boobies - liners

Class 1
Class 2
Class 3
Class 4
Class 5
Class 6
Class 7
Class 8
Class 9
Class 10
Class 11
Class 12

19. At what age do most babies need to start eating cereal? *6 months*

20. What is the father's role in breastfeeding? What are the advantages for him? (Father, please answer.)
- *support* *-portability* *-less work*
- *smell*
- *expense*

21. For the first few weeks after birth, what kind of care will the baby need?
- *umbilical cord care*
- *TLC*

22. What kind of care will the mother need?
- *TLC*
- *rest*

23. How many extra calories do you use each day while breastfeeding? *500*

24. What kind of a diet does a nursing mother need? *healthy nutrient dense*

25. What shouldn't a nursing mother eat? *greens may make baby gassy*
alcohol, caffeine, spicy foods, dairy?

26. Why are breast pumps rarely necessary? How are some of them dangerous?
body will react differently w/ baby & pump - different chemicals

27. Why is it best not to use breast pads most of the time? Which breast pads are the most dangerous?
ones w/ plastic - encourage bacteria

28. What would cause you to suspect you have a breast infection and what should you do about it?
- Pain, redness, fever, flu like symptoms, discolored, shooting pains

29. Should you stop breastfeeding on that breast if infection develops?
no
- increase salt intake to stop infection

30. Where can you get more information on breastfeeding and the working mother?
la leche league

31. When the time comes, what is the best way to wean from the breast?
gradually - one feeding at a time

white spots on babys cheeks/tongue = thrush & caused by yeast/sugar in diet

COMPLETE THIS SECTION AFTER YOU ATTEND A LA LECHE LEAGUE MEETING

32. What did you learn at the meeting?

33. What impressed you the most?

34. What questions will you ask while interviewing pediatricians?

35. What are the names and phone numbers of the La Leche League leaders in your area?

Thrush
2t apple cider vinegar to ½ c. water
2t baking powder to ½ c. water → apply to babys mouth & breast before & after feedings

STUDY HELPS

1. Why is what you eat more important than how much weight you gain?
   Different people gain different amounts of weight

2. According to Dr. Tom Brewer, what is the average number of pounds of weight gained by normal, healthy women during pregnancy? *35 lbs*

3. Why is good nutrition during pregnancy important for the baby?
   good for normal growth & development (p.16 each element)
   baby will pull nutrients from mom

4. Why is good nutrition during pregnancy important for the mother?
   healthy pregnancy
   less infection / discomfort
   more strength & stamina

5. At what time during pregnancy are the baby's brain cells growing and developing at their most rapid rate?
   8 months gestation

6. How does having good nutrition during pregnancy help to reduce the likelihood of:

   Toxemia (pre-eclampsia) – *75g + protein = 0% risk of toxemia*
   <75g = 44% increased risk

   PROM – *strong healthy membranes less likely to rupture*
   Premature rupture of membranes
   Hypovolemia and hemorrhage – *reduces likelihood*
   by providing nutrients needed for healthy blood volume

7. List food groups necessary for a well-balanced diet and the number of servings of each Dr. Brewer recommends.

8. What happens if you have all the food groups except one or two?
   unbalanced diet – body can't function properly

9. How does nutrition affect pregnancy, labor and birth?
   Strong healthy mom & baby

10. List things that may be important to avoid during pregnancy.
    mercury, drugs, smoking, alcohol

11. What is the best nutrition for most babies after birth?
    breastmilk

Class 1 Class 2 Class 3 Class 4 Class 5 Class 6 Class 7 Class 8 Class 9 Class 10 Class 11 Class 12

Class 1
Class 2
Class 3
Class 4
Class 5
Class 6
Class 7
Class 8
Class 9
Class 10
Class 11
Class 12

PREGNANCY

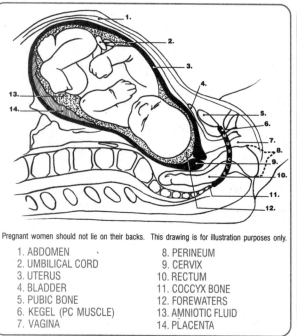

Pregnant women should not lie on their backs. This drawing is for illustration purposes only.

1. ABDOMEN
2. UMBILICAL CORD
3. UTERUS
4. BLADDER
5. PUBIC BONE
6. KEGEL (PC MUSCLE)
7. VAGINA
8. PERINEUM
9. CERVIX
10. RECTUM
11. COCCYX BONE
12. FOREWATERS
13. AMNIOTIC FLUID
14. PLACENTA

Abdominal breathing: moving air into and out of the lungs by movement of the diaphragm muscle, not the chest wall.

Braxton-Hicks contractions: (pre-labor or false-labor) normal intermittent painless uterine contractions, (last few months of pregnancy).

Contraction: shortening or tightening of the uterus.

Embryo: developing human baby the second through eighth week after conception.

Engaged/dropped: the entrance of the presenting part of the baby into the pelvis prior to birth.

Fetoscope: a stethoscope used to listen to (auscultate) the baby's heart beats and other sounds.

Fetus: the unborn baby between the ninth week and birth.

Gestation: growth of the baby from conception to birth while the mother supports and nourishes it.

Hyperventilation: over-breathing leading to an abnormally low level of carbon dioxide (CO_2).

Trimester: one-third portion of pregnancy, about three months.

Pregnancy can be a time of joy. It is important to widen your understanding of how your body works at this time. Learn how to work with the natural process to increase your comfort and safety. Learn how your body works and how you can work with your body.

It is important for coaches to learn about the physical and emotional changes that take place normally during pregnancy. This will help coaches to be more supportive, understanding and helpful.

GENERAL ASSIGNMENTS

☐ Tailor sit: often.

☐ Squat: often.

☐ Butterfly: (5) 1X a day.

☐ Pelvic Rock: (30) 4X + 60 at bedtime.

☐ Kegel: 150X a day.

☐ Walk 10 min + 5 min.

☐ Relax 10 min 2X a day.

☐ Fill out Pink Nutrition Worksheet.

☐ *Husband-Coached Childbirth*
    Read chapters 3, 4, 7, 12.

☐ Fill out *Student Workbook*, page 25.

☐ Arrange for Birth Place Tour: see page 101.

☐ Go to Student Center on: www.bradleybirth.com

MASSAGE

Discuss what kind of massage she enjoys. Talk about what feels good and helps to encourage deep relaxation. Many kinds of massage can be useful in labor. What kind of lotion, oil, or cream does she like? Experiment and find what works well for her. Be careful to avoid anything with a strong odor, as this is often distracting to a laboring woman. What parts of her body could you massage which would encourage relaxation? Try: her lower back, her feet, her legs, her shoulders, her arms, her hands, and her fingers. What kind of motion does she enjoy? Try: rubbing, scratching, tapping, stroking, but remember that these motions must convey relaxation. A good way to have her communicate what she likes is to have her demonstrate on you. Be sure to communicate openly about this both now and in labor so that you will know what she likes. Practice massage every day this week. Place your hands palm up, finger tips touching. Have her put her hand, palm down, on top of yours, then gently massage her hand starting at the wrist and circling your thumbs over and over again as you move down to her fingers. Massage each finger. Then stroke the surface of her hand. Do this to top and bottom of hand.

GESTATION

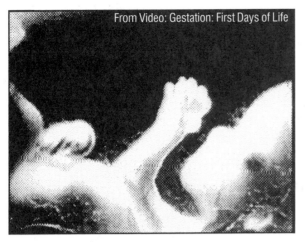

From Video: Gestation: First Days of Life

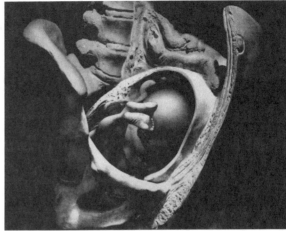

3 1/2 MONTHS -The baby is approximately 3 inches, weighing 1 oz., about 40,000 times larger than the egg from which it started. All organs are present, including a nervous system and heart which started beating 21 days after conception.

5 MONTHS - About 8 inches, weighing 1 1/2 lbs. The baby functions in this safe environment, moving and kicking. The baby is protected in many ways. 25% to 35% of babies are breech at this point. All but 4% will turn head down before birth.

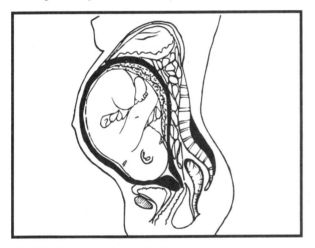

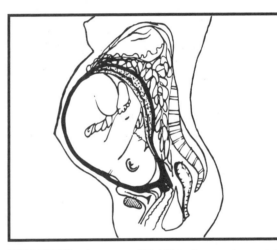

8 MONTHS - 6 pounds, 18-20 inches long. This baby has grown and developed until the mother's intestines, stomach, and lungs have a lot of pressure on them. Weight is being added at this time.

FULL TERM - Average of 7 1/2 to 9 pounds, and 20-21 inches long. Notice the difference in these two pictures. After baby drops or engages, the pressure is less on the mother's lungs, but greater on the bladder. The average length of gestation is 41 1/7 weeks, (with a range of normal between 36-44 weeks).

DRUGS DURING PREGNANCY

As Dr. Bradley explained in *Husband-Coached Childbirth*, if the mother weighs 140 lbs. and the baby weighs 7 lbs., the baby can receive twenty times the effect of a drug that the mother receives. This is a simplification. In fact, some drugs affect the baby more, some less.

Be careful. All of the following can reach and affect your baby during pregnancy: street drugs, prescription drugs, over-the-counter drugs, social drugs, natural drugs such as: teas, homeopathics, herbs, etc, food additives, household chemicals, and environmental hazards.

When considering using a drug during pregnancy, be sure to weigh the benefits and the risks.

YOUR BABY HAS A LOT OF BUILT-IN PROTECTION

Class 1
Class 2
Class 3
Class 4
Class 5
Class 6
Class 7
Class 8
Class 9
Class 10
Class 11
Class 12

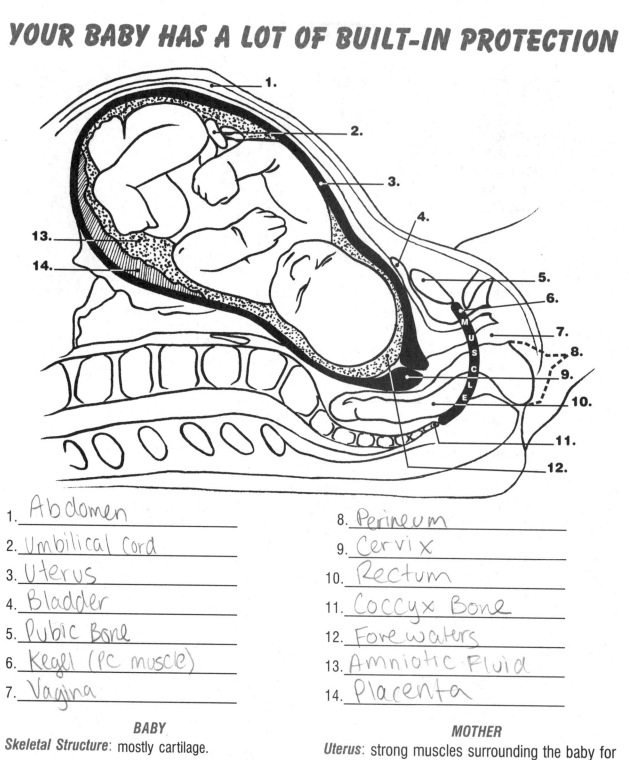

1. Abdomen
2. Umbilical Cord
3. Uterus
4. Bladder
5. Pubic Bone
6. Kegel (PC muscle)
7. Vagina

8. Perineum
9. Cervix
10. Rectum
11. Coccyx Bone
12. Forewaters
13. Amniotic Fluid
14. Placenta

BABY

Skeletal Structure: mostly cartilage.

Muscles & Skin: for support and protection.

Vernix: a creamy protection for skin to help with water environment.

Amniotic Fluid: to stabilize temperature & equalize pressures.

Bag of Waters: balloon-like structure; keeps contents together & germs out.

MOTHER

Uterus: strong muscles surrounding the baby for protection & process of pushing baby out at birth.

Pelvis: gives support, stability & protection.

Abdominal Muscles: provide protection & insulation.

Fatty Tissue: cushioning, temperature control & protection.

PC Muscle: support, encourages baby to put chin on chest at birth.

BEING COMFORTABLE IN PREGNANCY

Please check with your Healthcare provider about medical problems or anything you feel worried about. These ideas are hints other mothers have found helpful. Talk to your Bradley® teacher for further suggestions.

HEARTBURN
1. Identify offending food and avoid it.
2. Engage in moderate physical activity.
3. Eat apples, toast, papaya, or yogurt.
4. Try smaller meals; eat slowly.
5. Avoid carbonated drinks.
6. Walk after meals.

GAS
1. Identify offending food and avoid it.
2. Lie down and do abdominal breathing.
3. Do pelvic rocks.
4. Avoid carbonated drinks.

BLEEDING GUMS
1. Know that this may be aggravated by increased circulation (all mucous membranes are more sensitive during pregnancy).
2. See your dentist, have teeth cleaned.
3. Try increasing Vitamin C (oranges, etc.).

VARICOSE VEINS
1. Improve circulation.
2. Avoid standing in one position for prolonged periods.
3. Stay out of chairs, tailor sit on floor, change positions often and elevate legs frequently.
4. Do pelvic rocks.
5. Lie on couch on your side with feet up on couch arm or pillows for 5 minutes; follow with side relaxation.
6. Do ankle circles, not pointing toes, several times a day.

LEG CRAMPS
1. Try pelvic rock to improve circulation, squat, tailor sit, sleep with legs elevated slightly.
2. Avoid pointing toes or stretching too hard.
3. Check to see if salt intake is adequate.
4. Eat foods rich in calcium.
5. To stop a cramp in progress, point heel or stand on affected leg.
6. Check your diet.
7. Check exercise.

HEMORRHOIDS
1. Improve circulation; avoid constipation.
2. Do pelvic rocks.
3. Put feet up on small stool while on toilet for bowel movement.
4. Take warm sitz baths.
5. Do the Kegel exercise.
6. Increase fluids.

FATIGUE
(Normal in most cases but could be a sign of anemia, lack of water, or dehydration.)
1. Tune in to your body.
2. Get more rest.
3. Alleviate stress - take naps.
4. Cut hours, if working.
5. Don't overdo it - cut back on activities.
6. Maintain good nutrition.
7. Increase fluid intake.

CONSTIPATION
1. Eat lots of fresh or dried fruit (variety is important).
2. Drink lots of water.
3. Try high fiber foods.
4. Get daily exercise.
5. Avoid taking laxatives or straining while moving bowels.
6. Try putting low stool under feet while going to bathroom.

BACKACHE
1. Use good posture at all times.
2. Pelvic rock to tone muscles and improve posture.
3. Stand only for short periods of time.
4. Increase calcium.
5. Walk.
6. Soak in warm tub.

WEIGHT GAIN
1. Understand that there is no set weight gain which can be applied to all women.
2. Eat a well-balanced diet, including plenty of protein daily.
3. Avoid junk foods, fats, sugar.
4. Get lots of daily exercise (walking, swimming, bicycling, etc.).

©2010 AAHCC

SORE BREAST(S)
1. Wear a well-fitting cotton bra.
2. Apply heat.
3. Support breasts while lying down.
4. Avoid underwire bras.

SLEEPING PROBLEMS
1. Get enough exercise.
2. Cut out caffeine, sodas, etc.
3. Sleep with pillow supporting back and knees.
4. Have coach help to make climate more serene.
5. Naps may be necessary.
6. Warm beverage, milk or non-caffeine tea.

VAGINITIS (YEAST INFECTION)
1. Tailor sit.
2. Wear cotton panties or no panties at all.
3. Eat yogurt to help prevent yeast infection, especially if taking antibiotics.
4. Tell your birth team.
5. Wash hands prior to and after going to bathroom.

WATER RETENTION
1. Get daily exercise, but do not overdo it.
2. Increase protein intake; try Brewer's Yeast.
3. Remember, swelling may be a sign of a healthy pregnancy. Some swelling is normal.
4. Try adding more salt (may reduce swelling).
5. Drink lots of liquids, water, natural juices (cranberry, grape, etc.).
6. Eat fruits high in potassium, especially canta-loupe.

SHARP PAIN IN GROIN
May be cramping of the round ligament.
1. Do pelvic rocks.
2. Stop and lean forward until it goes away.
3. Take it easy and avoid jerky movements.
4. If it persists, call doctor.

MOODINESS
Know that this is generally due to hormonal changes, extra blood & fluids. It is common and considered normal. It may come and go.
1. Eat a piece of fruit.
2. Add high protein snacks to diet.
3. Change activity; do something fun.
4. Take a nap.

HEADACHES
1. Relax, especially facial muscles, and rest.
2. Be cautious about aspirin and Tylenol® (all drugs you take reach your baby).
3. Take a walk and/or nap and drink water.
4. Watch foods you are eating; may be an allergic reaction (MSG, pesticides, nitrates, caffeine, etc.).
5. Call doctor if they persist or are very severe.

PAINLESS RHYTHMIC CONTRACTIONS (BRAXTON-HICKS CONTRACTIONS)
These are generally good for you and baby; pre-labor warm-ups. Be prepared for remote possibility of early labor. If you are concerned, call your medical team.
1. Food or water may make a difference.
2. Change activity, rest.
3. Shower.
4. Do abdominal breathing.
5. Remember that these strengthen uterus, and help baby mature.

MORNING SICKNESS
This is generally caused by lowered blood sugar.
1. Eat fruit or protein.
2. Eat protein snack before retiring.
3. Eat dry crackers in morning before getting up.
4. Drink sparkling cider or juices.
5. Get lots of rest.
6. Eat small amounts frequently.

DANGER SIGNS:
Pregnancy is generally a very healthy time for most women. Pregnancy lasts only a short time and it is best to relax and enjoy it. Your body often knows best and tries to signal you if there is a problem. We suggest you tune-in to your body. The following are danger signs that you should be aware of. Call doctor immediately if you have:
1. Abdominal pain.
2. Vaginal bleeding.
3. Persistent vomiting.
4. Illness and/or high fever.
5. Painful urination or unusual vaginal discharge.
6. Sudden decrease in baby's movement or no movement.
7. Dizziness.
8. Persistent headache.
9. Excessive puffiness in hands or face (some swelling is normal).
10. Sudden, uncontrollable gush of water from vagina.
11. Anything coming out of vagina (bag of waters, umbilical cord, foot, hand, etc.).

COACHING CHALLENGES

TAKING CARE OF YOURSELF

1. What arrangements have you made so that you will be available during the labor?

2. Have you considered possible "false alarms"? How will that affect your arrangements at work?

3. How will "false alarms" affect you emotionally?

4. What will you wear during labor? Do you have an extra change of clothes if labor goes on for a long time or the bag-of-waters bursts all over you? Will you need to change into a scrub suit?

5. What shoes will you wear? Are they comfortable? Can you stand up in them for hours?

6. What additional toiletries will you need for yourself? (Suggestions: toothbrush, mouthwash, breath mints, shaving supplies, deodorant, swim suit for shower with mother.)

7. What food and drink will you bring for yourself? Will you take extra cash for vending machines or cafeteria? When will you pack these things? What if, for some reason, you don't bring any food or drink with you? Can someone get what you need?

8 What coaching aids will you need to have with you in labor?

9. What can you do to conserve your energy during labor?

10. What will you do if your partner is in active labor and she needs your full attention, but you need to go to the bathroom?

11. What can friends/family/back-up coach do for you?

• If you are going to a hospital that requires you to change clothes before entering the delivery room, change early; your wife will need you when the time comes.

• Her needs may change suddenly during active first-stage labor. She may not have the time to politely ask you to do something differently. She's likely to be very abrupt. Don't get offended. Be flexible. Remember, she needs to focus all of her energy on relaxation.

• Conserve your energy too. Get a chair to sit on. If the bed is big enough, lie down.

• Understand what is going on. Ask questions if you need to.

• Coaches need support and encouragement too. If you need some encouragement or some assistance, please call your Bradley® instructor. We care.

Class 1 | Class 2 | Class 3 | Class 4 | Class 5 | Class 6 | Class 7 | Class 8 | Class 9 | Class 10 | Class 11 | Class 12

whatit's *Choices* *pros/cons*

STUDY HELPS

1. Discuss the pros & cons of choices you may have:

Birth place:	Exams:
Cesarean:	Bed Rest:
Circumcision:	Admitting procedures:
Ultrasound:	Options:
Electronic fetal monitor in labor:	IV:

2. What exercises could you do for more comfort during pregnancy?

3. List ways the baby is protected while inside the mother's body.

4. List five things you like about your medical team:

5. What tests are normally done during pregnancy by your medical team?

6. List the steps you should follow when discussing issues with your medical team:

7. List several ways of monitoring the baby:

8. List three obstetrical devices which use ultrasound:

9. List ten things that relax you:

MOTHER	*COACH*
1.	1.
2.	2.
3.	3.
4.	4.
5.	5.
6.	6.
7.	7.
8.	8.
9.	9.
10.	10.

* Schedule Birth Place Tour- Discuss in Class 11, see page 101.

Class 1 · Class 2 · Class 3 · Class 4 · Class 5 · Class 6 · Class 7 · Class 8 · Class 9 · Class 10 · Class 11 · Class 12

THE COACH'S ROLE

→ effects on mind
demerol – through IV
less invasive than epidural may put you
may have a nightmare

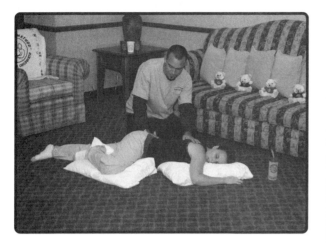

Analgesia: a chemical or drug agent that reduces the perception of pain without loss of consciousness; narcotic; relaxer (sic).

Anesthesia: a chemical or drug agent that blocks pain and may or may not cause loss of consciousness, permitting surgery or other painful procedures. *epidural – longer lasting*

Birth place: place where birth is planned to occur, or does occur. May be home, hospital, birth center or other place.

Birth team: medical professionals, family, friends and support persons selected by the family to share the joy and enhance the comfort and safety of their birth.

Medication: a drug, chemical or other agent used to relieve pain or treat disease.

Labor coach: husband or other supportive person selected by mother to assist in preparation for and the act of birthing.

Motivation: motivating or being motivated; to give impetus to; to incite; to impel.

Natural childbirth: as our great-great grandmother gave birth; childbirth regarded and performed as a natural process without analgesia, anesthesia or surgery.

Nursery: the department in a hospital where newborn babies are cared for.

Coaches function before and during the birth. They are essential in the physical preparation of the body during training, long before the birth. They also prepare the athlete's mind so that there is a clear conception and understanding of the tasks involved. By their interest and enthusiasm, they should be living symbols to the spirit of the player, motivating the individual to want to play the game at her best.

In most cases, the father is the BEST coach; but, if this is not possible, a coach who is dependable and can relate to the mother works well. Additional coaches or doulas may be helpful as back-up, but should not replace or interfere with the family.

MENTAL RELAXATION

Now that you have mastered several techniques to achieve physical relaxation, we will begin working on the next step, mental relaxation. Mental relaxation has to do with what you are thinking about. You will need to find a relaxing poem, story, or some relaxing music to use as you practice and to bring with you in labor. Once your partner is in a comfortable position and has become physically relaxed, calmly read to her or turn on the music and strive to achieve an even deeper level of relaxation. What other things could you read or recite to encourage relaxation? This week, work on finding poems, prayers, stories, or music that could be useful, and then try them out. Put together your own collection in a notebook, file, or on a recording. Many women like this technique because when they concentrate on the music or story, time seems to pass more quickly.

GENERAL ASSIGNMENTS

- ☐ Tailor sit: often.
- ☐ Squat: often.
- ☐ Butterfly: (7) 1X a day.
- ☐ Pelvic Rock: (40) 4X + 80 at bedtime.
- ☐ Kegel: 150X a day.
- ☐ Walk or exercise: 10 min + 10 min a day.
- ☐ Relaxation practice: 15 min 2X a day.
- ☐ Praise and encourage each other.
- ☐ *Husband-Coached Childbirth*: chapter 5.
- ☐ Nutrition
- ☐ Go to Student Center on: www.bradleybirth.com

Class 1 Class 2 Class 3 **Class 4** Class 5 Class 6 Class 7 Class 8 Class 9 Class 10 Class 11 Class 12

THE COACH NEEDS TO BE:

ENTHUSIASTIC

"The loving encouragement from a trained coach can do more for the comfort and relaxation of his wife than any amount of medication." Dr. Robert A. Bradley. How well you do your job will directly affect how much pain the mother will experience and how well the labor will go.

1. How can you enthusiastically encourage the mother to do her exercises and have good nutrition every day?

2. Why is the above important?

3. What ways can you communicate your enthusiasm?

COMMITTED

The goal of achieving an unmedicated birth is an important and impressive one. Your commitment is essential.

1. Why do you feel it is important to have a natural birth?

— healthy for the baby /mom

— quicker recovery

2. Reasons breastfeeding is important to the coach: *(write down others that apply)*
   - *Sleep*
   - *Smell*
   - *Portability*
   - *Health of mother & baby*
   - *Expense*
   - *Convenience*

3. These are the "Whams" described in *Husband-Coached Childbirth*.
   - *Ill effects of drugs on baby.*
   - *Prolonged labor.*
   - *Interference with Breastfeeding.*
   - *Effect of nursery on baby.*
   - *Effect on Mom.*
   - *Unjoyfulness.*

4. What other effects could medication have?

5. Things to look for when choosing a pediatrician.
   - ☐ Recommendations from others.
   - ☐ One who will work with you.
   - ☐ Takes time to answer all your questions.
   - ☐ Respects your opinions/decisions.
   - ☐ One who realizes that YOU are ultimately responsible for the care of your baby.
   - ☐ _____

STRONG

1. What strengths do you bring to this pregnancy?
    Coach: Mother:

2. What strengths does your partner bring to this pregnancy?
    Coach: Mother:

UNDERSTANDING

"Since the mind is closely linked to the body, the physiological changes in a pregnant woman's body affect her mind in certain subtle ways. As her constant companion, you should know and understand these ways and adjust your way of thinking and acting accordingly. Your job is more than just planting the seed. You must now tenderly nurture it, cultivate it properly, and not let the weeds of anxiety, self-doubts, or unresolved hostilities spring up. Pregnant women, coached by natural childbirth oriented husbands, sparkle with the joy of life. The little nuisances of physical discomfort from their enlarging abdomens are joyfully taken in stride as necessary nuisances without becoming all-encompassing." *Husband-Coached Childbirth*

1. Do you understand what she is going through?

2. What more could you do to help her during this challenging time?

3. Have you read *Husband-Coached Childbirth*?

A RELAXATION EXPERT

Relaxation is the key to labor in The Bradley Method® and can be very helpful, even for women who have not practiced much prior to labor. But, it is the couple who has really mastered the techniques taught in class who can realize fully the incredible benefits of deep relaxation in labor.

1. Where does your partner tense up first?

2. What helps to relax her?

3. Three types of relaxation:
    •*Physical*   •*Mental*   •*Emotional*

4. Are you working together every day on relaxation? ❏ *YES*

5. How can you help to alleviate stress in your lives?

Class 1 | Class 2 | Class 3 | **Class 4** | Class 5 | Class 6 | Class 7 | Class 8 | Class 9 | Class 10 | Class 11 | Class 12

WHAT COACHES OFTEN SAY

Fill in the blanks.

FIRST STAGE LABOR

1. "Concentrate on your hands being loose, and ___limp___, and ___relaxed___."

2. "Take ___one___ contraction at a time."

3. "The stronger the contraction, the more you ___relax___."

4. "You're doing a ___great___ job."

5. "Each contraction brings us ___closer___ to the birth."

6. "I want you to completely ___relax___ with this next ___contraction___."

breathe into a tight place

7. "Isn't my wife doing ___awesome___!"

8. "Picture your cervix ___opening___ like a ___flower___."

9. "The discomfort in your back means that the baby is moving ___down___."

10. "Think about the baby moving ___through___ your ___pelvis___."

11. "You're doing _____."

12. "You look ___beautiful___."

13. "I love ___you___."

14. "Think of yourself as a leaf floating on a ___pond/lake___."

15. "Let ___go___, give ___in___ and let your baby come out."

learn how to let go / surrender / don't fight the pain

SECOND STAGE LABOR

16. "Hold your breath as long as is ___comfortable___."

17. "Push to the point of ___comfort___."

18. "You're doing ___great___!"

19. "___Great___ job! "

20. "I can see the ___head___."

21. "___Baby___'s almost here."

22. "Completely ___relax___ between ___contractions___ and recoup your energy."

23. "I'm so ___proud___ of you!"

24. "We ___did___ it!!!"

25. "I ___love___ you ... and our baby!"

©2010 AAHCC

DRUGS, MYTHS AND BIRTHING

by Jay Hathaway, AAHCC

The medical journal *Epidemiology* reported in October 2000, that adult drug addiction is linked to the administration of drugs during labor to their mothers. Other reports have linked adolescent suicide to birth events.

I believe that this is only the tip of an iceberg of problems caused by the liberal and unnecessary epidemic of narcotics given to pregnant women by medical professionals with the best of intentions during childbirth.

If your teenager took heroin or cocaine you would be plenty mad, and very worried... right? Is it possible that there is a connection between teenage drug abuse and mothers who chose drugs for pain relief during birth? There is very little difference between heroin, morphine, demerol, nisentil, stadol, nubain, sublimase, codeine, fentanyl, oxycontin, oxycodone or even, methadone. All of these are opioids, like opium. There is precious little real difference at all. In equi-analgesic dosages (that is, to produce the same amount of pain-relief), they share the same side-effects.

What is the difference between cocaine and the drugs used for epidurals, etc.? Precious little, too. In fact, they all end with the same suffix, marcaine, bupivacaine, nesacaine, chloroprocaine, carbocaine, mepivacaine, sensorcaine, lidocaine, novocain, xylocaine all of them... caines just like cocaine. All these drugs belong to the same chemical family.

Robert Bradley, MD, led the fight against these drugs for over forty years, with mixed success. While nearly 90% of Bradley Method® births are drug-free, most other-method or non-method births are not births at all, but drugged deliveries. The rate of drugged babies at birth in the U.S. today is about 90%.

OK, you ask, what right has a man got to discuss drugs? He never experienced birth... Ah, but I did get born didn't I? The old saying "If men had babies there wouldn't be any babies" might be true. But, I have helped train over four thousand families to give birth, and have helped train over three thousand Bradley® teachers most of whom are also Bradley® parents. I have witnessed and photographed over 150 births and have discussed this topic with literally thousands of families. Marjie and I have six children, three by "knock-em-out, drag- em-out" obstetrics, and three by The Bradley Method®. I have shared the pain and the joy of natural birth, and the pain caused by drugs.

I have come to believe that a group of erroneous beliefs are popular today:

> *MYTH ONE*: Childbirth pain is unbearable and pointless.
> *MYTH TWO*: Childbirth drugs work. That is drugs can help make childbirth pain-free, or at least less painful.
> *MYTH THREE*: Childbirth drugs are safe for the mother.
> *MYTH FOUR*: Childbirth drugs are safe for the baby.
> *MYTH FIVE*: Drugs are given when the mother needs them most.
> *MYTH SIX*: Pain is better if delayed.
> *MYTH SEVEN*: Childbirth drug administration is painless.
> *MYTH EIGHT*: It hurt so bad, even with the drugs that I must warn everyone to insist on plenty of drugs. Just imagine how bad it would have been without the drugs!

MYTH ONE: **Childbirth pain is unbearable and pointless.**

Every female member of your family tree beginning with Adam and Eve, right down to your grandmother, or great grandmother had a Bradley® birth. Natural childbirth was all there was... back then, and only in the last few generations was unnatural childbirth even a possibility. Drugs for delivery began in the 1840's. Cesarean section is not an ancient operation. This major surgical operation has been done on living mothers for little more than a century. The majority of births today, worldwide, are natural, often due to lack of medical personnel or facilities, and many of the countries which lack our sophistication seem to produce bumper-crops of kids.

Birth is not without pain. Birth is never without risk, this may be even truer lately as the U.S. currently ranks 29th in worldwide infant mortality (*Pediatrics*, Jan. 2010).

Could it be possible that pain is not all bad? Could pain have any purpose? Why is it there? Pain can be minimized, rearranged, changed or postponed... but I doubt it is ever truly gone. The saddest thing about obstetrical anesthesia may be... if it works, it robs the mother of feeling the birth.

Natural childbirth works! This may sound radical, but it is true. Not only does it work, but it has a purpose... perhaps it is better to do it right... in the first place.

Class 1
Class 2
Class 3
Class 4
Class 5
Class 6
Class 7
Class 8
Class 9
Class 10
Class 11
Class 12

The Bradley Method®

Class 1
Class 2
Class 3
Class 4
Class 5
Class 6
Class 7
Class 8
Class 9
Class 10
Class 11
Class 12

MYTH TWO: Childbirth drugs work. That is, drugs can help make childbirth pain-free or at least less painful. Arnold Bresky, MD, said at a recent Bradley® teacher training that in labor, women make noise, and he was trained to make them quiet by giving them drugs to "shut-them-up".

Several years ago a couple in our classes had returned to share their birth experience. The husband explained without reservation that his wife had "needed" to take some Demerol® (a narcotic) during labor because of the pain, his wife interrupted him and said "Honey, you don't understand, that medication did nothing for the pain! ...all it did was shut-me-up!"

Has silence been mistaken for pain relief? I started thinking about this issue and asked Marjie for her personal opinion. She had had Demerol® for our first three children. She said it differently, but the idea was similar... she said the drugs had not made the pain go away. In fact, they seemed to make pain worse. She felt she could no longer "handle" the pain, lost a sense of time, etc... If Demerol® causes sleepiness, the mother's rest periods seem to disappear, making labor appear to be continuous.

So, I started asking women who had medicated deliveries a new question: "Did the drugs work?" And I was amazed at the answer, often it was "No! " Of the hundreds of women I have asked, the vast majority report that the medication did not "work" on them. The strange thing is that often they are convinced that they are somehow different, they are often amazed that anyone else shares their experience of this myth. Especially disturbing accounts often came from mothers who did not learn any of the many natural, effective techniques for handling pain in labor because they expected the drugs to "work" and assumed they would feel no pain. By the time they realized the drugs were not going to render their labors painless, they were helpless to do anything else.

MYTH THREE: Childbirth drugs are safe for the mother. Item: *Wall Street Journal*, August 24, 1983 "FDA Issues Warning On the Use of Local Anesthetic For Pregnant Women". It seems that 16 American women had died from epidural anesthesia using .75% bupivicaine.

Victor Berman, MD, said at a recent Bradley® teacher training: "All drugs used in childbirth are dangerous, all of them are poisons. If they are given a little bit more than they should be, they have serious effects. If they are given a little bit more than that, they will have disastrous effects on both the baby and the mother, probably to a greater extent on the baby. And even in so-called small or normal doses, every now and then somebody turns-up that is more sensitive than the average person and there is some horrible result. The over-use of drugs, or the over-sensitivity to drugs is associated with such things as cerebral palsy, brain damage..."

MYTH FOUR: Childbirth drugs are safe for the baby. All obstetrical pain killing drugs have been proven to reach the unborn baby, including epidurals. (*Anesthesiology* 29: 951) A recent study reveals that epidurals and even so-called locals "may result in significant neonatal drug exposure." (*Am. J. Obstet. Gynecol.* 149:403) All doctors know this, but many parents do not. The American Academy of Pediatrics, Committee on Drugs has stated that there is no drug, either by prescription, over-the-counter or food additive that has ever been proven safe for the unborn baby. All childbirth pain medications, "relaxers", and anesthetics do reach the unborn baby, usually within one minute. The myth of the so-called placental barrier is long-since dead. Dr. Bradley said for decades that this so-called barrier is nothing more than a bloody sieve, and now we have scientific proof that he was right.

As I have explained, most drugs used in childbirth are narcotics. One of the first effects of narcotic drugs is respiratory depression, making it harder for the baby to begin to breathe. The short-term dangers of drugs are well known, but the long-term effects are more subtle. For years mothers have been told their babies are "a little sleepy" from receiving drugs. Perhaps this is more of a threat than was suspected earlier. A study in the *New England Journal of Medicine*, September 1985, of cocaine addicted mothers said that street drugs made the babies passive and "If the infant is passive, the mother becomes resentful and passive... ." Epidural, spinal and "local" anesthetics use "caine"- type drugs. "Caine"-type drugs can lead to child abuse by parents, these experts conclude. How can street "caines" be bad but, medically administered "caines" be harmless? The chemical effects of drugs are the same, regardless of the source or the intentions of their administrators.

A study of Demerol® from *Anesthesia Analg.* :64, 1985 showed "Even low doses of Demerol® may adversely affect neonatal behavior." They went on to say "The effect was still apparent at three days of age." A news article from *United Press International* (January 14, 1979) reported an average loss of four IQ points per child, leading to a national loss of fourteen million IQ points a year is caused by pain-killing drugs used in childbirth.

MYTH FIVE: Drugs are given when the mother needs them most.

People often refer to "the discomfort of labor and the pain of delivery." They presume that, although labor (first stage) is uncomfortable, the real pain is during delivery (second stage). I have asked hundreds of women who had given birth without drugs the following question: "If you had your labor to do over again, knowing what you now know, and there really existed a completely safe and effective way to relieve you of all sensation, what part of your labor would you want to use it for?" Almost without exception women reported that although they might be tempted to go through hard labor without sensation, they would never want to miss the sensations of giving birth to their babies. For the majority of mothers, portions of their *labor* are perceived as being considerably more painful than the *actual birth*. Most also added that although their labors were uncomfortable and at times quite painful, they felt there was a purpose to their pain and that because they worked so hard for their babies they felt they loved and appreciated them more.

Only the mother knows how much pain she is in. Some women actually handle their pain by grunting, screaming, or making noises. They should not be given drugs just to quiet them down. Often, a woman asks for drugs if the stress of labor becomes overwhelming during transition (which only lasts a short time). The call for drugs may actually be a cry for support and encouragement rather than for narcotics. With some loving emotional support, the birth happens soon; naturally, joyfully.

MYTH SIX: Pain is better if delayed.

Many years ago I heard a talk by Herbert Ratner, MD, during which he stated that drugs took the pain out of labor *where it belongs* and delays it until after the baby comes, *where it does not belong*. Think about it, no matter how painful the labor or birth, the pain is usually *before* the baby comes out. After the birth the mother is able to concentrate her attention on the baby and the process of mothering. Drugs have to be detoxified by mother and baby, and may leave both recipients less able

to function optimally. An epidural or spinal may relieve the pain before the birth but it can leave the mother paralyzed and in pain for hours *after* the birth, and sometimes with a headache that can last for days or longer.

MYTH SEVEN: Childbirth drug administration is painless.

Many mothers have told me "The drugs hurt worse than having a baby." Remember: the drugs have to get into the body somehow, and rarely is it painless.

Demerol® or it's cousins are injected through a needle or an intravenous line (another needle). The majority of anesthetics are administered into very sensitive areas of the body with very long needles indeed. The epidural or spinal is actually injected into the interior of your spine. Paracervical and pudendal block anesthesia are actually injected deep inside the area around the vagina. This type of "pain-relief" can actually be quite painful.

MYTH EIGHT: It hurt so bad, even with the drugs that I must warn everyone to insist on plenty of drugs. Imagine how bad it would have been without the drugs!

A lot of things in life are painful, and yet, nobody uses anesthetics for them. Ever see the face on a marathon runner, or a tri-athlete? Ever watch a football player get tackled... pain! Ever watch a baseball player crash into the center-field wall to catch a dumb little ball and save the game? They don't ask for drugs... oh, a few of them have tried to do this stuff while taking drugs... and guess what happens... a loser is born. Drugs decrease performance. What have you ever done that could be more important than giving birth? Drugs mess-it-up.

How can we change the societal "knowledge" that birth is awful? Each of us must share the JOY of birth with everyone we can... friends, neighbors, acquaintances, and best of all... our children.

After giving birth yourself, become a Bradley® teacher. If you can give birth, perhaps you can help others regain the JOY of birth. This world needs more Bradley® births.

The Bradley Method®
Box 5224, Sherman Oaks, CA 91413-5224
(818)788-6662
www.bradleybirth.com

Class 1 | Class 2 | Class 3 | Class 4 | Class 5 | Class 6 | Class 7 | Class 8 | Class 9 | Class 10 | Class 11 | Class 12

CLASS 5 *(week 5 of 12)*

INTRODUCTION TO FIRST STAGE LABOR

Class 1
Class 2
Class 3
Class 4
Class 5
Class 6
Class 7
Class 8
Class 9
Class 10
Class 11
Class 12

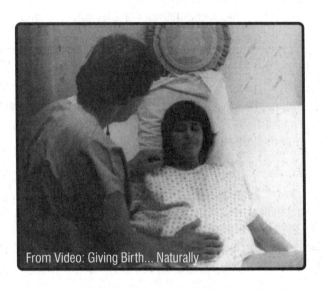

From Video: Giving Birth... Naturally

Anterior presentation: presenting part of baby is rotated so the occipital bone of the baby (back of the head) is toward the front of the mother, most common presentation.

Bag of waters: the membranes that surround the baby and the water in the uterus; BOW; amnion is inner layer, chorion is the outer layer.

Birth canal: vagina.

Centimeter: a unit of length, approximatley 2.5 centimeters per inch. One penny is 2 cm in diameter.

Cervix: "baby door"; the neck of the uterus; the lower end of the uterus.

Dilation: opening; the act of opening the cervix to approximately 10 cm.

Effacement: thinning; the act of thinning the cervix, expressed in percentage.

Natural alignment plateau: (NAP); the normal period in many labors when dilation is not increasing, but uterine activity continues. Often ends with rapid complete dilation.

Prep: may include: shave, enema, blood pressure measurement, blood sample, history, etc..

Bloody show: passage of blood tinged mucous or mucous plug prior to onset of labor, or in labor, there is no fixed time before labor begins.

A woman's body is designed to labor in preparation for birth. The average time of uninterrupted, rhythmic contractions is approximately 15-17 hours, but may vary greatly. Although there may be many bouts of pre-labor, real labor ends with the birth of a baby.

Every woman is special, and there are many variations of labor length and strength. These classes are designed to educate you in the natural process of labor and to teach you the many safeguards that nature provides to protect the mother and baby at this time. This usually generates the confidence needed to birth naturally.

GENERAL ASSIGNMENTS

❏ Tailor sit: often.

❏ Squat: often.

❏ Butterfly: (10) once a day.

❏ Pelvic Rock: (40) 4X + 80 at bedtime.

❏ Kegel: 200X a day.

❏ Walk: 15 min. + 10min. a day.

❏ Relaxation: 15 min. + 20 min. a day.

❏ Nutrition

❏ *Husband-Coached Childbirth*: chapter 6.

❏ Go to Student Center on: www.bradleybirth.com

STROKING

As your partner concentrates on relaxing and letting go, put your whole hand at the back of her neck and slowly but firmly stroke down across her shoulder, upper arm, elbow, forearm, hand, and fingertips. As you are using this technique, reinforce it verbally by telling her to concentrate on relaxing completely in response to your touch. Talk about stroking the tension down and out of her body. This technique can be used on her arms, legs, back, and face. Practice all of these. This technique can be used any time in labor and is especially good to use late in labor if it is becoming harder to relax. If at some time in labor she is experiencing a lot of pain, has been disturbed, or feels as if she cannot go on, try this stroking, coupled with a lot of encouragement. Guide her through one contraction at a time and remind her that every contraction brings the baby closer.

HOW YOUR BODY WORKS

Watch changes to the cervix, bag of waters, descent of baby's head, and the angle of the uterus.

Class 1
Class 2
Class 3
Class 4
Class 5
Class 6
Class 7
Class 8
Class 9
Class 10
Class 11
Class 12

1. How your body works to prepare for labor.
   - Practice (Braxton-Hicks) contractions — *entire abdomen tighter*
   - Increased blood volume
   - Relaxin & Hyaluronidase — *hormones*
   - Colostrum & Immunities
   - Soften Cervix
   - Mucous plug
     might be bloody

eat, drink, sleep, shower

may feel bodyaches up to week before

2. How your body works in early first stage labor.
   Note: When a mother lies on her back and the uterus moves forward during a contraction, gravity pulls it down causing a great deal of pain.
   - Contractions
   - Hunger
   - Thirst
   - Diarrhea
   - Dilation
   - Effacement
   - Station
   - Bloody show

3. How your body works during active first stage labor.
   - Powerful contractions
   - Continued thirst
   - Loss of modesty
   - Loss of appetite
   - Need to urinate often
   - Continued dilation & effacement

4. The Natural Alignment Plateau (NAP). *25-30% of moms experience*
   Contractions may continue - dilation stops for a while.
   Possible reasons:
   - Physical alignment
   - Softening of cartilages
   - Balancing of hormones
   - Production of immunities for baby
   - Certain muscle groups needing a break
   - Every woman is different and prep-time of birthing system will vary.

★ move around change positions

DILATION / TIME graph — N.A.P., AVERAGE

4 THINGS MEASURED DURING VAGINAL EXAMS

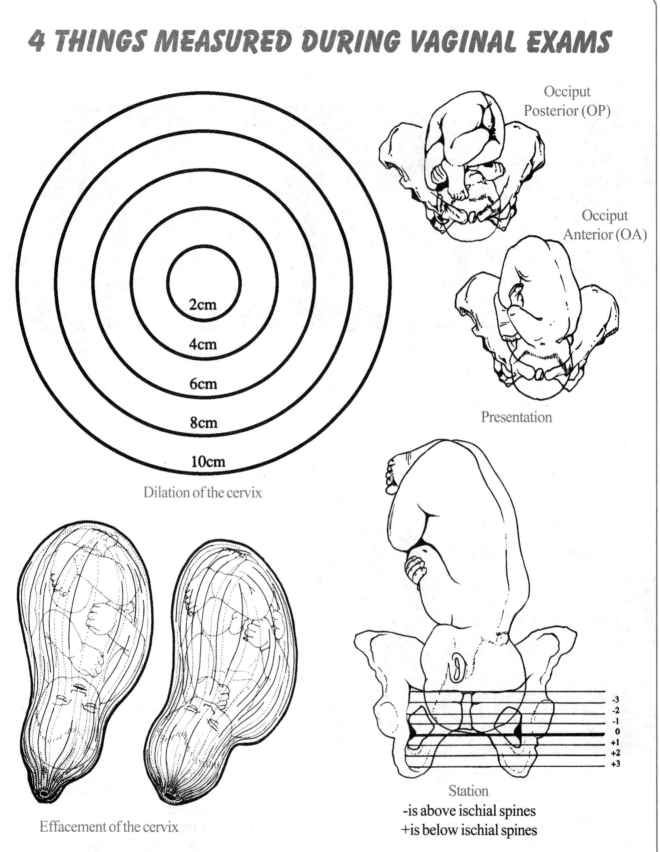

2cm

4cm

6cm

8cm

10cm

Dilation of the cervix

Occiput Posterior (OP)

Occiput Anterior (OA)

Presentation

Effacement of the cervix

Station
-is above ischial spines
+is below ischial spines

-3
-2
-1
0
+1
+2
+3

Class 1
Class 2
Class 3
Class 4
Class 5
Class 6
Class 7
Class 8
Class 9
Class 10
Class 11
Class 12

1. Possible drawbacks associated with vaginal exams: pre-mature rupture of membranes, risk of infection, discomfort of mother, possibly misleading information, increased chance for a cesarean, etc.

2. Some doctors recommend against having vaginal exams: routinely or if the bag of waters has broken.

FIRST STAGE PRACTICE

Natural Abdominal Breathing

Breathing is a natural, normal part of life and regulates itself according to the needs of your body every minute of your life, including labor. Abdominal breathing is the type of breathing that is normal for humans.

BENEFITS OF ABDOMINAL BREATHING

1. It's natural.
2. Uses less energy.
3. Lowers blood pressure.
4. Conducive to relaxation.
5. Self-regulating.
6. Uses capacity of the lungs.
7. Avoids hyperventilation, which may be dangerous.

EFFECTS OF CHEST BREATHING

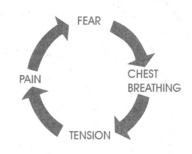

FEAR → CHEST BREATHING → TENSION → PAIN →

Timing Contractions

A first stage contraction is like a wave building up in intensity, staying hard for a while, then subsiding. The peak is generally reached by 30 seconds. Even in a long contraction, it does not generally get harder after 30 seconds. It may stay hard for a while, but it does not get harder before subsiding. Contractions are generally timed from the start of one to the start of another.

SAMPLE TIMING

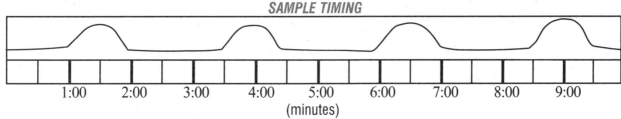

1:00   2:00   3:00   4:00   5:00   6:00   7:00   8:00   9:00
(minutes)

1. *How far apart are these contractions? (frequency)*

2. *How long are these contractions lasting? (duration)*

3. *When do the contractions peak?*

4. *When is the next contraction likely to begin?*

When You Practice

Every day, from now on, after working for ten minutes on your relaxation techniques, go through a series of five practice contractions. Contractions should be two minutes apart and last sixty seconds each. Follow these guidelines as you practice.

MOTHER'S CHECKLIST	COACH'S CHECKLIST
Sleep imitation - eyes closed	• Check her position.
• Do not move during a contraction.	• Check her relaxation.
• Abdominal breathing.	• Rub her back.
• Relaxation.	• Simulate contractions*.
• Face relaxed.	• Guide her breathing.
	• Time contractions.
	• Talk to her.
	*Simulate contractions during practice only.

Think about how your body will be working as you practice. Take one contraction at a time. Concentrate on each contraction as it builds up in intensity, stays hard for a few seconds and then gradually subsides. The stronger the contraction, the more you relax.

OVERVIEW OF LABOR AND BIRTH

These are general guidelines to help you follow the course of a normal labor. Remember that *every labor is different* and these are only guidelines. It is possible for a labor to begin at any of these points, skip stages, or seem to move back and forth between stages with no clear definition.

STAGE	EMOTIONAL SIGNS	BEHAVIOR	PHYSICAL SIGNS	
EARLY FIRST STAGE	First emotional signpost: **Excitement** "Maybe this is it! ...But then I'm not sure."	"Putsy-Putsy." Anxiously cleaning, talking, walking, smiling. Walking is important. Many mothers feel restless and need to walk. She may or may not want to move or talk during contractions. She may be hungry.	She may have bloody show (mucous plug, spotting of blood-tinged mucous or mucous discharge) runny nose, several bowel movements, need to urinate frequently. Note: if heavy bleeding occurs, call birth attendant.	
FIRST STAGE	*Acceptance* "This is it." Confident and committed. "This is a lot of work, but I can do it."	Tries various positions and techniques to find what works best and is most comfortable for her. Walking is still important. Looks as if she is working hard but usually prefers to keep busy between contractions.	May be hungry depending on how long the labor has been. May be able to talk and/or move during contractions, but it is an effort. She feels many changes occuring in her body and is settling into a pattern.	
LATE FIRST STAGE *(Hard Labor)*	Second emotional signpost: **Seriousness** The "do-not-disturb" and "get to work" attitudes.	Losing modesty. May still need to walk, but uses slow deliberate movements. May need to lie down. Appearance of sleep, deeply concentrating. May like sitting on the toilet.	No longer hungry. No longer talkative, even between contractions. She may be sweating, bag of waters may break, she becomes uncomfortable if disturbed, tenses up, or needs to urinate.	
TRANSITION	Third emotional signpost: *Self-Doubt* "This is so hard. I'm so tired. I can't take any more. I give up." *Surrender*	Confused, unsure, scared, nervous, may want to go home, may move around a lot, may give up, may yell at you, may be handling things fine.	May be sweaty, shaky, hot then cold, nauseous, may vomit, burp, have cold feet. Bag of waters may break if it hasn't yet.	
SECOND STAGE	*Calmness* and *Determination* Desire to complete the task. "I want to hold my baby."	No longer modest. Either gradually or suddenly gets urge to push. Usually more alert and may become more talkative between contractions. May be very tired and might sleep between contractions.	Mucous discharge and some bloody discharge, bag of waters may break if not broken, if it breaks during a contraction, water may burst all over the place. She seems to have gotten a second wind.	

Class 1 · Class 2 · Class 3 · Class 4 · Class 5 · Class 6 · Class 7 · Class 8 · Class 9 · Class 10 · Class 11 · Class 12

CONTRACTIONS	SENSATIONS	NEEDS	REMINDERS
Generally 10 minutes apart or less, lasting 45 - 60 seconds and becoming progressively stronger and closer together. Generally do not space out from changing activity.	Strong contractions that peak at about 30 seconds. Possible pressure or cramping feeling. It generally feels better to walk around and keep busy. She may notice many changes in her body during this time.	Keep busy and don't become too excited. This may or may not be actual labor. Have someone with you. Eat if hungry, drink often, get some rest if at all possible.	Walking helps to open the inlet of the pelvis. Adrenalin can slow or stop the labor. If labor stops, don't get discouraged. Rest, eat and go on. This happens often.
Contractions are becoming stronger and more frequent. Generally five minutes apart or less lasting around 60 seconds.	Increasing pressure and fullness in pelvis, backache, cramping feeling across lower back or as menstrual cramps. May feel stretching in pelvis with sore pubic bone. Pelvic rocks may help.	Support and reassurance. She should not be separated from her coach from now on. Freedom of movement, plenty of space and fresh air are often important. Timing contractions helps.	Conserve your energy, you don't know how long you will be in labor. It is often good to do something fun and entertaining to help pass the time between contractions.
Intense and close, sometimes one on top of another. Generally (but not always) follow a regular pattern and last 60 seconds or more. May put pressure on bladder causing need to urinate during contractions.	Hard work, intense, almost overwhelming, you lose track of time, you must concentrate on staying relaxed, tensing up causes pain. Tremendous pressure in pelvis. Feels good to relax completely between contractions and to rest.	Dim lights, comfortable temperature, freedom to move around, peaceful environment, drink and go to the bathroom often. It is important to "give in" and allow the labor to take over.	This is it! You are doing it! Relaxation is the key. Remember the natural alignment plateau. Labor is much more than mere dilation. Be patient, you and your baby need this time.
May become irregular, may double peak, may come one on top of another, may stop completely for a while.	Sensations change greatly often causing panic, disbelief, and fear. You may feel the baby shifting into alignment with pelvis, a lot of pressure down low. This may be hardest part. It will soon be time to hold your baby.	Reassurance, encouragement, good coaching, various relaxation techniques. Do Not Disturb! Take one contraction at a time. Avoid drugs, the hard part is almost over.	Remember: Transition may be the hardest part, but it doesn't last long. The baby is coming soon. Your baby is counting on you!
Change to expulsive type. May ease into stage by only pushing at peaks or get sudden urge to push. Usually more time between contractions now.	Wait for overwhelming need to bear down. Generally feels better to push and hurts if you don't. Feels sort of like having a huge bowel movement. Most mothers feel a stretching and burning feeling which builds to a tremendous release as baby is born.	Encouragement and freedom to choose best position. May need a quick lesson in how to push. Everyone do as mother asks. Give her ice chips or water and remind her to completely relax between contractions.	There are many pushing positions. Squatting and classic are most efficient. Push to point of comfort hold breath only as comfortable. This stage can last a few minutes or many hours. Happy Birth-Day!

Class 1
Class 2
Class 3
Class 4
Class 5
Class 6
Class 7
Class 8
Class 9
Class 10
Class 11
Class 12

Class 1 Class 2 Class 3 Class 4 **Class 5** Class 6 Class 7 Class 8 Class 9 Class 10 Class 11 Class 12

ASSISTANT COACHES (DOULAS)
Read and utilize Assistant Coach's Manual

Some couples like to have one or more people at the birth assisting the coach or watching siblings. Read *Children at Birth* if siblings are present. These people might be family, friends or a paid assistant. Here are some ideas to make this effective. Birth is not a spectator sport!

Assistant Coach Role:
Assist the coach.
Take care of siblings if present.
Stay positive and enthusiastic.
Respect this family and their decisions.

Preparations:
(Discuss your specific role with the parent's personal choices.)
Will assistant coach be present:
during vaginal exams, while mom is in the bathroom, during the birth, if a complication arises, etc.?

Pack a Bag:
1 or 2 changes of clothes.
Swim suit if coaching in shower.
Personal toiletries.
Food.
Phone numbers and change or phone card.
Mobile phone.
Camera, film, etc.

Make Necessary Arrangements:
Time off work.
Babysitting.

Information - Read and attend Bradley® classes if possible:
General - 1st stage, 2nd stage, 3rd stage.
When is it "time"! - see workbook.
Important in labor - mothers generally like: walking, drinking, and using the bathroom often. See B.E.S.T. article.
If baby comes out without medical people present, catch, call for help (911), make sure baby is breathing, leave cord alone, put baby to mother's breast immediately, and put a blanket over the two of them.
Be ready for - a lot of hard work, noises moms can make in labor, discharge, bag of waters breaking, blood, pain, and placenta.

General Jobs for You:
Be positive and enthusiastic - smile!
Maintain a relaxed environment - quiet, calm.
Keep sipper bottle filled and ready.
Keep records - a journal, timing contractions, interesting things that happened.

How the Assistant Coach Might Help At Home - Early Labor:
Set up peaceful environment.
Handle phone calls.
Wash the dishes.
Prepare food.
Keep her sipper bottle filled.
Prepare for the Birth-Day party.
Gather last minute things.
Change the bed and leave the house clean.

If Moving:
Prepare the car - towels or underpads, pillows, full sipper bottle, basin, her bag, her I.D., insurance card, workbook.
You may be asked to drive the car.

Active Labor:
Be sure coach is eating and drinking regularly.
Be friendly and speak softly as people come in. Say "Isn't she doing great!"
Handle telephone - update family regularly Say "These things take time."
Praise and reassure her - she needs to hear it.
Rub her feet or hold and stroke her hand.
Get cool wash cloths - refill her sipper bottle.
Rub the coach's shoulders.
Take over if he needs a bathroom break.
Keep track of contractions, positions, bathroom, etc.
Take pictures if they want.

Do whatever you can to help the coach so he can focus on the important job of helping the mother.

Be ready to do a lot of the less glamorous "behind the scenes" type work.

Be aware that you may be asked to step out for a while. Some of labor can be very private.

STUDY HELPS-REVIEW

1. How will having had good nutrition affect how your body works in first stage?

2. How does having done your exercises affect how your body works in first stage?

3. How does being calm and relaxed affect how your body works in first stage?

4. How does adrenalin affect how your body works in first stage?

5. What are the causes of adrenalin production in first stage?

6. How does your position affect how your body works in first stage?

7. What role does the bag of waters play during first stage?

8. What effect does medication have on how your body works in first stage?

9. How does dehydration affect how your body works in first stage?

10. What are the typical prepping procedures at your birth place?

Note: See Page 125 for examples of First Stage Labor Positions

Class 1 Class 2 Class 3 Class 4 **Class 5** Class 6 Class 7 Class 8 Class 9 Class 10 Class 11 Class 12

CLASS 6 *(week 6 of 12)*

INTRODUCTION TO SECOND STAGE LABOR

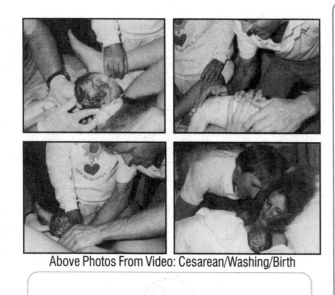

Above Photos From Video: Cesarean/Washing/Birth

Afterbirth: the placenta and membranes expelled after the baby is born.

Apgar rating: named for Dr. Virginia Apgar, a rating of the baby's condition, 2 points each for: heart rate, respiration, muscle tone, reflexes and color.

Episiotomy: surgical incision made in perineum.

Fetal Heimlich maneuver: natural phenomenon, as baby is born, mother's intact perineum pushes inward below the baby's rib cage... expelling mucous from baby's mouth and nose.

Ischial spines: bony prominences at lower edge of pelvis (narrowest point of pelvis) serves as measuring point of baby's descent, point called zero station.

Perineum: the skin and tissues between the vagina and the anus.

Physiological (positive) pushing: mother-initiated pushing, only to the point of comfort, holding breath only as long as comfortable, tuning-in to her own bodies instructions and urges.

Station: the downward progress of the baby relative to the ischial spines expressed in cm. i.e.: -1, +2, etc.

If your body is in good condition (low risk and no medication), your body tends to push effectively, causing the baby to rotate, squeezing the baby (which gets rid of fluids), stretching the perineum and delivering the baby. Generally, the head is down, then to the side, and finally, after head is born, faces up (looking at mommy). Third stage is the process of expelling the placenta by contraction of the uterus.

Most births can be accomplished without medication or interference. The time required varies greatly, depending on the circumstances. A well-nourished mother who follows the low-risk program takes advantage of how well designed and efficient a pregnant woman's body is during birth. Birth is certainly a miracle.

GENERAL ASSIGNMENTS

- ☐ Tailor sit: often.
- ☐ Squat: often.
- ☐ Butterfly: (10) once a day.
- ☐ Pelvic Rock: (40) 4X + 80 at bedtime.
- ☐ Kegel: 200X a day.
- ☐ Walk: 15 min 2X a day.
- ☐ Nutrition
- ☐ Relaxation, labor practice: 20 min 2X a day.
- ☐ Read "Choices" in *Children at Birth*.
- ☐ *Husband-Coached Childbirth*: chapter 8-10.
- ☐ Go to Student Center: www.bradleybirth.com

MUSCLE OBSERVATION

For each muscle group, have the mother tense and then relax a little, then a little more and finally completely relax. Work to achieve this "complete relaxation." Coach, feel the difference between the tension and each step toward complete physical relaxation. While she's completely relaxed, massage her and reinforce this positive accomplishment. You are learning now about the various degrees of physical relaxation. As the coach, you need to learn to recognize not only the difference between tension and relaxation, but the difference between partial relaxation and complete physical relaxation. Continue to practice this until the mother feels she has memorized the feeling of being deeply relaxed and you can easily tell whether she is completely relaxed or not. Practice every day this week and use this deep relaxation in labor so that you can avoid unnecessary pain.

Class 1 Class 2 Class 3 Class 4 Class 5 Class 6 Class 7 Class 8 Class 9 Class 10 Class 11 Class 12

HOW YOUR BODY WORKS

Be aware of the bag of waters, the descent of the baby, and the rotation the baby goes through.

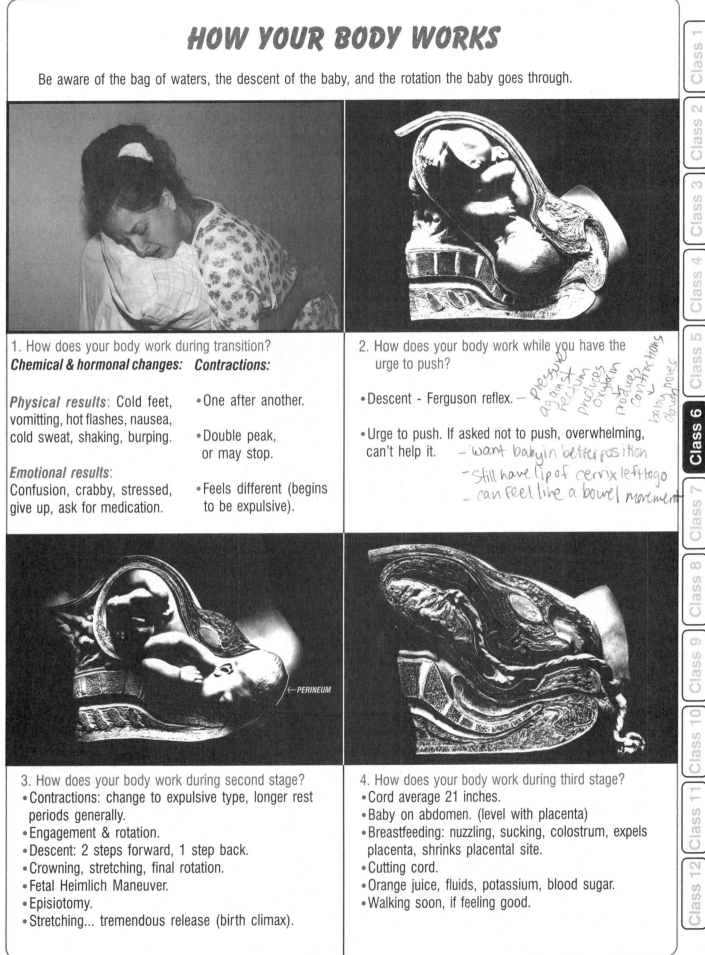

1. How does your body work during transition?

Chemical & hormonal changes:

Physical results: Cold feet, vomitting, hot flashes, nausea, cold sweat, shaking, burping.

Emotional results: Confusion, crabby, stressed, give up, ask for medication.

Contractions:

• One after another.

• Double peak, or may stop.

• Feels different (begins to be expulsive).

2. How does your body work while you have the urge to push?

• Descent - Ferguson reflex. — *pressure against rectum produces oxytocin produces contractions baby moves down*

• Urge to push. If asked not to push, overwhelming, can't help it. *— want baby in better position — Still have lip of cervix left to go — can feel like a bowel movement*

← *PERINEUM*

3. How does your body work during second stage?
• Contractions: change to expulsive type, longer rest periods generally.
• Engagement & rotation.
• Descent: 2 steps forward, 1 step back.
• Crowning, stretching, final rotation.
• Fetal Heimlich Maneuver.
• Episiotomy.
• Stretching... tremendous release (birth climax).

4. How does your body work during third stage?
• Cord average 21 inches.
• Baby on abdomen. (level with placenta)
• Breastfeeding: nuzzling, sucking, colostrum, expels placenta, shrinks placental site.
• Cutting cord.
• Orange juice, fluids, potassium, blood sugar.
• Walking soon, if feeling good.

Class 1 Class 2 Class 3 Class 4 Class 5 **Class 6** Class 7 Class 8 Class 9 Class 10 Class 11 Class 12

Class 1
Class 2
Class 3
Class 4
Class 5
Class 6
Class 7
Class 8
Class 9
Class 10
Class 11
Class 12

TRANSITION

Transition is like the shifting of gears between first and second stage. It usually occurs after many hours of active labor when the contractions follow a regular pattern and you've established a routine.

Transition can come on suddenly or gradually. Occasionally, a mother will drift back and forth between active labor and transition. Active labor usually lasts many hours, but transition is generally relatively short, perhaps 10 to 30 minutes.

Please list the possible signs of transition.

Not everyone has a tough transition, but if you are coaching a woman who does, you are going to need to know these very important points.

ATTITUDE

Stay calm, confident and reassuring. Don't let this take you by surprise. You are well-prepared. You know what to expect and you know how to handle it. This can be a challenging phase, so remember your training. She may not be confident at this time, but you will be. Your remaining calm, confident and reassuring will help her more than anything else.

Keep a positive attitude. Transition is a good sign. You've reached a major milestone. Congratulations! Your hours of labor are almost over; it's almost time for the birth. Though right now you may feel unsure, concerned, scared, or tired, you must remain confident and in control. This phase will not last long. Soon you'll begin second stage, assist your partner during pushing, begin to see the baby's head, witness the birth, and hold and touch your new baby.

Remember, transition is normal. This is not an indication of medical emergency or complication. If there is anything medically wrong, your birth team will alert you. If they haven't said anything about it, then assume everything is fine physically, and concentrate on transition as an emotional challenge.

At this time she is likely to say things like, "I can't do it anymore. I give up." This is good; she's surrendering her struggle to be in control. Her labor will soon be over. Surrender is an important part of the birth process.

How would this affect you and what can you, as the coach, do to better prepare yourself for this challenge?

ACTIVITY

Stand up. Show her that you've recognized her need for additional support and that you're on top of things. Take an active role. Guide her through contractions and, if necessary, tell her what to do every step of the way.

Take one contraction at a time. Think about this contraction only. Don't be concerned about whether you or she can handle any more. Can you handle this one? Okay, then, do it! This may be her last first stage contraction and second stage will be a whole different situation.

Assist her in any way you can. Some women need a lot of verbal coaching at this time, others tell you to "shut up." Some women need a lot of massage and touching, others say, "Don't touch me!" Don't get offended, just find what you can do to help her and do it. Remember to use the techniques that you've practiced for so long. They can be especially helpful now.

What techniques can you use, even if she does not want you to talk to her?

What techniques can you use, even if she does not want to be touched?

What important things are you responsible for, even if she will not let you talk to or touch her at all?

UNDERSTANDING TRANSITION

1. She may feel out of control, but that's understandable; She does not control the labor.

2. She may feel tired, but that's understandable; she's been working very hard, and she will soon get a burst of new energy.

3. She may feel confused, upset, and unsure, but transition is the time of confusion, it will soon pass.

4. She may not know what to do anymore, but that's understandable and that's why she has you.

5. She may say it really hurts, but that's understandable; she's having a baby! Soon the baby will be born and it will all have been worth it.

6. She may cry, but that's understandable; she's going through a very emotional time, but she has your shoulder to cry on and your strength to see her through.

7. She may say she needs "something for the pain," but that's understandable; transition is the most common time for women to ask for medication. You know how to help her through without drugs; you are the "something" that she needs.

8. She may criticize you, but that's understandable; she's in transition and she knows that you will not be offended.

9. She may think that she's not doing a very good job, but that's understandable; she is going through a time of self-doubt. Labor is such a big challenge, it is never exactly what you expected. She needs you to remind her what a good job she's doing.

10. She may say that she really wants the drugs, but that's understandable; transition can be difficult, but it does not last long. By the time the medication might take effect, transition would probably be over and she won't want to miss the wonderful sensations and feelings of accomplishment that come from giving birth without drugs.

• *Transition is sometimes the most difficult part of labor.*

• *Transition does not last long.*

• *Hang on.*

• *Your baby will be born soon.*

• *You can do it!*

Class 1
Class 2
Class 3
Class 4
Class 5
Class 6
Class 7
Class 8
Class 9
Class 10
Class 11
Class 12

SECOND STAGE PRACTICE

Second Stage Basics:
- Push to the point of comfort.
- Hold your breath as long as is comfortable.
- Choose the most comfortable position.

PUSHING

Although, by the end of pregnancy, the uterus is generally strong enough to push the baby out without your help, most women feel an overwhelming urge to push with their contractions. Women should tune-in to their bodies and push to the point of comfort. The strength with which women need to push will vary during second stage. Often, the urge to push decreases considerably as the baby crowns so that mothers can gently push the baby through, lessening the chances of tearing or needing an episiotomy.

BREATH HOLDING

You do not have to hold your breath, although most women need to use it as a means of pain control. Holding your breath traps a cushion of air which helps the uterus move forward and keeps the baby in the proper alignment with the pelvis. It also increases intra-abdominal pressure. Mothers should tune-in to their bodies and breathe whenever they feel the need to.

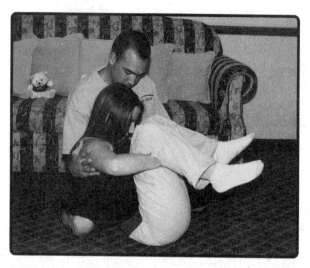

Classic position - This is the most common and one of the most effective pushing positions. Practice this once or twice until you feel comfortable with it.

Note: It is not necessary to practice 2nd stage positions a lot... because your body will be much different, and these positions will be much easier to assume during the birth.

Pushing with the third breath, helps to push closer to the peak of a contration, unless the urge is sooner.

The following is a description of how you might handle a second stage contraction.
(Do not actually push during practice.)

MOTHER	COACH
• Take first deep breath; exhale. Then a second breath; exhale. Then take third deep breath; push; hold it only as long as is comfortable.	• Assist her into her pushing position.
• Pull your legs back(with elbows up and out).	• Remind her to: push to the point of comfort, hold her breath only as long as comfortable, open up, push down and out.
• Put your chin on your chest.	• Watch her perineum during contractions (it should be bulging).
• Relax the rest of your body while you push.	• Make sure that her face, shoulders, legs and feet are relaxed as she pushes.
• To take another breath, tilt your head back, exhale completely, take a fresh breath, put chin on chest. Do as often as needed during each contraction.	• Have her completely relax between contractions. Give her ice chips and a cool washcloth.

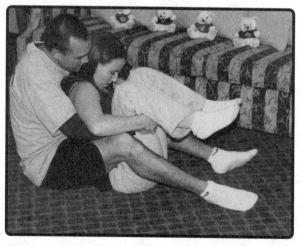

Alternate Classic Position - This alternative is generally more comfortable and gives the mother better support. If this position would be applicable in your situation, practice until you feel comfortable with it.

SECOND STAGE POSITIONS

Although the classic position is the most common pushing position used, there are many other positions to choose from. Whatever position a woman chooses, there are certain basic guidelines for effective birthing.

1. Knees back with elbows up and out—this shortens the vagina and lessens the tension on the perineum. Speeds up second stage, reducing pain and burning sensation.
2. Chin on chest—closes the glottis, increases intra-abdominal pressure, aligns baby and uterus with pelvis.
3. Curved spine (do not arch your back)—so that the baby can come through the pelvis.

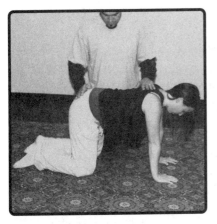

Side Position - Mother lies often on her left side, bringing up her knees and holding her top leg. This position enables the mother to have more control. Many midwives like this position and feel it helps avoid an episiotomy.

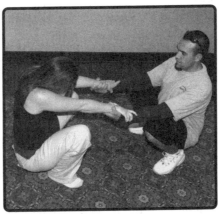

Squatting Position - Gives the mother great control over the birth. It is suggested for women who are in good condition and can squat well. It is also an emergency position used to bring down babies that are difficult to deliver.

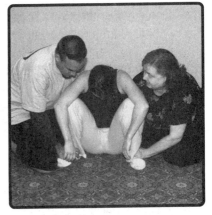

Assisted Squatting Position - Has the same benefits as the squatting position. One or two coaches can help to support the mother so that she feels more stable while pushing.

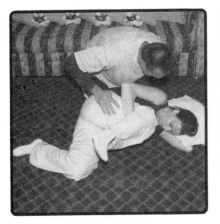

Hands and Knees Position - Like the pelvic rock position with the mother on the hands and knees. It is especially good for persistent posterior babies. The hands and knees position allows fluids to flow away from the baby's mouth and nose at birth.

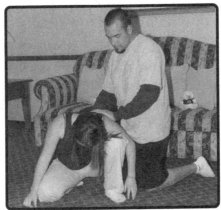

Asymmetric Position - Mother assumes a kneeling position with one knee down. She can switch from left knee down to right knee down between contractions. This is especially helpful for mothers who have a rim or lip of cervix.

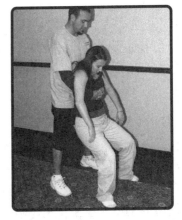

Standing - Mother stands and bends her knees slightly. She needs to be careful not to arch her back. This position is rarely used but it is a good birthing position and allows the mother to help catch the baby.

Class 1
Class 2
Class 3
Class 4
Class 5
Class 6
Class 7
Class 8
Class 9
Class 10
Class 11
Class 12

SECOND STAGE

1. List four things that will help you to recognize the urge to push.

2. What could you do if your partner is not fully dilated or has a lip of cervix left, but feels the need to push?

3. Women in labor often forget what they have learned. Please write a brief lesson on how to push.

4. Remember the mother's instincts are usually right; help her to follow them. How will you encourage your birth team to assist you to do what the mother feels is best?

5. How can you tell if the mother is relaxing the Kegel muscle while she is pushing?

6. What agreement do you have with your birth team regarding episiotomy?

7. What is your role if you are trying to avoid an episiotomy?

8. What is your role if a pressure episiotomy is going to be done?

9. Will you help to catch the baby? If so, who will be assisting the mother?

10. Who will cut the cord and when will it be cut?

11. What benefits are there to breastfeeding right away?

12. What can you do to take advantage of the sensitive period of bonding?

13. How and when will you get the mother some orange juice? Why is it important?

14. Where and when can the mother walk soon after birth? Why is this important?

15. How soon can the mother eat? How will you get her some food?

• *Second stage lasts an average of 2 hours, though it can be as short as a few minutes or longer than eight hours and still be normal.*

• *Squatting is the most effective pushing position because it opens the outlet of the pelvis by more than 10%.*

• *The first couple of hours after the birth are the sensitive bonding period.*

• *There is so much going on at the time of birth that it may take you a while to put things into perspective. Joy may be combined with fatigue, exhilaration with sorrow, and excitement with responsibility. Just let things settle. It is possible and normal to have mixed feelings.*

STUDY HELPS

1. Remember the natural alignment plateau? Could a mother who is only 4 centimeters dilated be going into transition?

2. What do the changes in the mother's body during transition cause her to experience, emotionally?

3. Most of the time, at what point does the bag of waters break spontaneously?

4. What role does the bag of waters play during second stage?

5. What causes the mother to feel the urge to push?

6. Under what conditions should a mother "lean into" the contraction?

7. What effect does the mother lying on her back have on how her body works in second stage?

8. What position causes the outlet of the pelvis to open 10-15% more?

9. What is the average length of second stage for a first-time mother?

10. What side-effect can occur if the mother pants or blows even through one contraction, at this point?

11. What is the importance of the fetal Heimlich maneuver?

12. What is an episiotomy?

13. When are episiotomies necessary?

14. Can episiotomies be done without medicating the mother and the baby?

15. What is the importance of putting the baby to the breast immediately after birth?

Class 1
Class 2
Class 3
Class 4
Class 5
Class 6
Class 7
Class 8
Class 9
Class 10
Class 11
Class 12

CLASS 7 *(week 7 of 12)*

PLANNING YOUR BIRTH

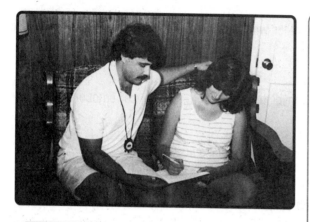

Amniotomy: artificially breaking the bag of waters.
Birth plan: a written plan expressing the family's desires in a normal birth, and also for possible complications.
Complication: a variation from normal birth which carries an increased risk. Some are relatively minor (posterior or breech), some are major (prolapsed cord, hemorrhage).
Consumerism: an approach to childbearing wherein the parents take the active decision-making role, with the active support and consultation of carefully selected medical professionals.
High risk: any condition of pregnancy which creates a higher than normal risk.
Informed consent: the act of agreeing to a medical procedure after receiving information regarding it's benefits, risks and weighing them and making up your own minds.
IV: intravenous, administration into a vein.
Low risk: a normal pregnancy, may have many variations but remains within normal risk range.
Positive communications: being able to express your preferences and decisions in such a way as to retain the enthusiastic support of your birth team.
Realistic expectations: recognizing the inherent risk of childbearing and the irreducible hazards. Also being realistic about what kind of support you can expect to receive from the birth team and birth place you have chosen. Accepting the normal variations in labor and birth regarding time, work and pain.

The kind of pregnancy, labor and delivery our children experience has a profound and lifelong effect on their health, including their mental and emotional health. On many issues (or interventions), even experts cannot agree. This places the challenge of decision-making directly on the parents' shoulders. Knowing the issues, and the pros and cons, can make a difference.

This section will help you to become aware of the choices available and help you to decide what things are important to you. Make a realistic birth plan to encourage you to have good communications with your birth team so you can work together toward the goal of the safest and most positive experience possible. For the majority of well-trained women, allowing labor to follow the natural course is the best and safest route. Medications and other interventions, such as cesarean sections, may be lifesaving in specific circumstances, but always have their own special additional risks. Labors should be evaluated on an individual basis, not as routine. Machines cannot replace good personal care.

GENERAL ASSIGNMENTS

- ☐ Continue nutrition and exercises.
- ☐ Write out procedures/choices.
- ☐ Birth plan step 2 - do alone, then share.
- ☐ Relaxation Practice - 20 min 2X a day.
- ☐ Walk 20 min +15 min a day.
- ☐ Labor practice - every day.
- ☐ Nutrition
- ☐ *Husband-Coached Childbirth*: chap. 11, 13, 14.
- ☐ Complete Breastfeeding Questionnaire - page 17.
- ☐ Student Center: www.bradleybirth.com

POSITIVE EXPECTATIONS

Work through your birth plan and make all the arrangements necessary as you prepare for your labor and birth. Then write a realistic story together, of your target birth experience. Include as much detail as possible. Make it a normal, realistic progression including the appropriate sensations, people, places, etc. Be sure that it is positive and reassuring. You will probably re-work your story several times, and that's fine. Every day this week, read the story to the mother when she is deeply relaxed. Then have her sit up and discuss her feelings. Did any part of the story make her feel tense, upset, uncomfortable? If so, you still have some things to work out. You could also write a story from the coach's point of view. This does not guarantee that you will have this target experience, but it will help you both feel more confident and tranquil about what you are likely to face.

MAKING PLANS FOR LABOR AND BIRTH

This section was designed to help responsible, healthy parents plan for a natural labor and birth. Positive cooperation between everyone involved is important. These plans should be made with the assumption that the labor will be normal and uncomplicated. If something out of the ordinary does occur, these plans may have to be changed depending on the situation at the time.(Bring copies to class for everyone to review & have copies at your birth.)

STEP 1. *Know your options* - Consider your many options having to do with: the rest of your pregnancy, labor, birth, and postpartum. Think about the choices you can make now, and the choices you will have to make at the time. You will discuss many options in class. Make a list of all your options. This list should include many things that you would choose during a normal labor and birth including: Where will your baby be born? When will you go to your birth place? Will you and your coach ever be separated? What prepping procedures will you go through? How will the baby be monitored in labor? Will you be free to move, walk and change positions as you feel the need? Will there be time limits on the length of your labor or pushing stage? What positions might you use in second stage? How will you push? Will you have an episiotomy? Will you take pictures? Will you breastfeed the baby immediately? Who will cut the cord and when will it be done? Will the baby ever be taken from the parents? When will you go home if you are at a hospital or birth center?

STEP 2. *Examine your feelings* - The mother and the coach both need to decide what things are important to them, and then discuss their feelings and make any compromises necessary.

STEP 3. *Consider your priorities* - List your choices in order of importance (most important first).

STEP 4. *Evaluate your situation* - Are your choices realistic? Are most of your preferences openly supported by your birth team? If not, will you compromise or make other arrangements?

STEP 5. *Meet with your medical professionals* - Make an appointment for both the mother and coach to talk with the doctor or midwife. Before that meeting, read the page on positive communications in this book and determine which of your choices your birth team and birth place normally support. Then make a brief list of the options you still need to discuss. At the meeting, start by explaining why you think they are special and why you've chosen them to support you during this very special time in your lives. Tell them what you've been doing to stay healthy and low risk. They are likely to be impressed that you've been actively working toward a positive and safe birth experience. Next, in a positive way, state your preferences that apply during a normal, uncomplicated labor and birth. Give your birth team a chance to state their feelings and the reasons for them. Finally, discuss emergencies and find out how your care provider would recommend handling such situations. Note your birth attendant's feelings and any changes you make. Thank them sincerely for their openness.

STEP 6. *Prepare for a positive experience* - Write up your final birth plan including your highest priorities. This final version of your birth plan should be used to set the tone for your labor and birth. Be careful to phrase things in a positive and polite way rather than making it just a list of demands. This can help everyone to feel more confident and increase your chances of having the birth experience you want.

STEP 7. *Be flexible* - A beautiful birth experience is important and will have a positive effect on the family which can last a lifetime. However, the health and safety of mother and baby come first. If an emergency does occur, crucial decisions affecting their lives and health must be made quickly, and will require cooperation, as you and your birth team work together.

Class 1

Class 2

Class 3

Class 4

Class 5

Class 6

Class 7

Class 8

Class 9

Class 10

Class 11

Class 12

What are your preferences during a normal labor, birth and postpartum period?

STEP 1 KNOW YOUR OPTIONS	STEP 2 MOTHER'S FEELINGS	COACH'S FEELINGS	STEP 3 LIST PRIORITIES

STEP 4
RE-EVALUATE
(if necessary)

STEP 5

OPTIONS WE WOULD LIKE TO DISCUSS REGARDING NORMAL LABOR AND BIRTH	POSSIBLE COMPLICATIONS WE WOULD LIKE TO DISCUSS WITH OUR MEDICAL TEAM

Class 1
Class 2
Class 3
Class 4
Class 5
Class 6
Class 7
Class 8
Class 9
Class 10
Class 11
Class 12

SAMPLE BIRTH PLANS:

A

We are very pleased with our choice of Dr. Smith and Anytown Hospital for our upcoming birth-day party.

We are well-prepared and educated and have done everything we can to stay healthy and low risk during this pregnancy. We are looking forward to a beautiful, natural birth and would appreciate all of the kind, encouraging care that you can provide.

Since this is a very special event in our lives, we have some preferences which may be different than your standard routine. We respectfully request that you consider our wishes and do not offer medication to us during labor unless an emergency arises. We also feel strongly that we (the mother and coach) remain together at all times during labor and that our baby be handed to us immediately after birth for breastfeeding and bonding.

We will, of course, be flexible on all these points if a complication does arise. Although we feel confident that everything will go normally, we trust that you will inform us if any problems come up so that we can discuss the choices to be made and come up with a new plan of action. We take our responsibility of being good parents very seriously and want to do what is best for our baby.

Thank you for your kind attention. We look forward to sharing this, one of life's most miraculous events, with the very special people on your staff.

B

In striving for as normal and peaceful a birth experience as possible, we request the following:

Time to labor.

Privacy during this intimate event.

Support from our labor assistant.

Freedom of movement both in and out of the bathtub or shower.

Flexibility on our part as well as our birth team's.

Positive Encouragement at all times, keeping in mind that labor and birth are natural processes at which we can marvel and must always respect.

Note: Example A is from a couple going to a traditional Dr. and hospital. Example B is from a couple going to a birth center. Your birth plan will of course be unique and reflect your preferences and your personalities.

STEP 6
OUR FINAL BIRTH PLAN

Your birth plan is a very helpful document expressing the desired outcome for you, your baby and those you have chosen to be part of this miraculous experience. Try and express to those involved with this birth helpful instructions on what you want this process to be. Now is the only time you have to make it very clear to the birth team your desires, wants, and dislikes. Your birth-team should be honored to be a part of your once-in-a lifetime opportunity. This will only happen once for you and this baby. Have a very Happy Birth-Day!

Positive Birth Plan Phrases

1. We are looking forward to having a natural childbirth. Please don't offer us any pain medication. We will let you know if we need it.

2. We are hoping to avoid needing _medication/ episiotomy_.

3. It is very important to us that _____, please help us in any way you can.

4. Please understand, we feel very strongly about _bonding w/ baby right after_ _____.

    Solution focused

5. We are looking forward to _____.

6. It would be helpful if you could _____.

7. We would like to avoid _____.

8. These are our preferences in the case of an uncomplicated labor. If a complication does arise, we will, of course, do whatever is necessary to keep mother and baby safe.

    In the case of a C-section
    Desires:
    Newborn Procedures:

Please prepare your birth plan and make copies for everyone involved in this event. Make sure to make extras to hand-out to nurses and/or last minute guests. Bring several copies to class 8 to share with the class to get positive feedback.

Class 1
Class 2
Class 3
Class 4
Class 5
Class 6
Class 7
Class 8
Class 9
Class 10
Class 11
Class 12

POSITIVE COMMUNICATIONS

AND GOOD RELATIONSHIPS ARE IMPORTANT TO A GOOD BIRTH EXPERIENCE.

Giving birth is a very emotional experience, and you need to be able to communicate with your medical team. Do not take for granted that they know what is important to you and your family.

1. Attend Bradley® classes and read *Husband-Coached Childbirth* so you know which choices are most important to you.
2. Coach and mother should set aside time and talk over each other's needs and expectations.
3. Make a special appointment with your doctor, telling the secretary that you want time to talk.
4. Coach and mother together, should sit and talk with the doctor, face to face.
5. Explain what things are important to you and why.
6. Your medical team is concerned about your safety and emotional needs. You must let them know what your needs are and how they can help you.
7. Show them a copy of the *Student Workbook* and assure them you are willing to work hard to be well-prepared.

CREATE POSITIVE FEELINGS AT THE HOSPITAL

1. Introduce yourself. Ask for (WRITE DOWN) your nurse's name. You may wish to send a Certificate of Appreciation after the birth.
2. Show your Coach Card and point out instructor's name.
3. Take the initiative in setting the atmosphere YOU want (chatty and relaxed or more calm and quiet).
4. Use positive comments and phrases; it will rub off. (e.g. "My wife is doing GREAT and is really working well with her contractions, isn't she?" "We are having GOOD strong contractions now.")
5. When the nurse is positive or supportive, verbally compliment her. It encourages repetition.
6. Ask questions in a direct, positive way. Make requests pleasantly. Try not to demand. Request more information. Say, "Will you help me?".
7. Give the nurse any information you have regarding the labor (loss of plug or water, pattern of contractions, back pressure).
8. Appreciate suggestions, whether or not they are applicable. Remember your training. The staff may not be totally knowledgeable in the Bradley Method®. You are. ("Thank you for your suggestion, I can take it from here." or, "Thank you for your suggestion; we tried it, but this works better.")

9. Be sure ALL requests are agreed to before you go into labor, so you are not arguing or upset with the hospital staff and doctor at this time. Iron these things out during pregnancy. Getting upset in labor ruins the experience for everyone.
10. Coaches, be positive and self-confident. It encourages a supportive attitude. Ask for needed information when entering the hospital (locations of blankets, ice chips, bathroom).

INFORMATION TO OBTAIN FOR INFORMED CONSENT IF A PROBLEM ARISES

Every situation is unique. Education in advance gives you background information, but information about specific problems can only be obtained at the time. Relax and ask for help understanding the situation. Speak up if you need more information or disagree. (i.e. everyone thinks you are too tired to continue and you disagree. Tell them! "I feel like I still have lots of energy. I want to continue.") The following questions should help the couple obtain the information they need to make wise decisions.

1. "Tell me more about this drug or procedure. Explain the reasons this is the best drug or procedure for me and my baby."
2. "What are the expected results? Will my baby and I be healthier for taking it or having it done?" (Is it a routine procedure?)
3. "Are there other options?"
4. "Tell me more about the known side effects and liabilities." (You might like to read the package insert if it is a drug.)
5. "Will its benefits outweigh the side effects?"
6. "What is the risk to me and my baby if I don't take it or have it done? Can we wait a while longer before deciding?"
7. "Could we have a moment alone to discuss this?"
8. "What procedures will also be done if we choose the procedure in question?" i.e.: Internal Continuous EFM, I.V. fluids, Restriction of movement and position, etc.

The Bradley Method®

PACKING CHECKLIST
WELL BEFORE YOUR DUE DATE:

1. Attend all your Bradley® classes; continue until you give birth.

2. Tour hospital and check out back-up for emergency situations.

3. Choose a health-care provider for your baby; interview several.

4. Arrange for baby-sitting and household help, if needed.

5. Pack your bag, these are typical items:

(handwritten note: — applesauce?? — whole grain toast w/pb = gatorade)

IN THE CAR:
- ❑ Puddle pads
- ❑ Pillows (with plastic bag under pillow case)
- ❑ Small basin
- ❑ 2 old towels (large & clean)
- ❑ Blanket (clean)
- ❑ *Student Workbook*
- ❑ Full gas tank (keep car above 1/2 tank last 2 months)
- ❑ Car seat (Infant/convertible)

FOR MOTHER:
- ❑ Husband/Coach
- ❑ Nightgown
- ❑ Lightweight bathrobe
- ❑ Old slippers
- ❑ Nursing bra(s)
- ❑ Honey and spoon or honey straws (absorbed quickly into blood stream, faster than sugar)
- ❑ Warm socks
- ❑ Plastic trash bag
- ❑ Your own pillow with plastic bags under colored pillow cases to help identify your pillows
- ❑ Hair ribbon
- ❑ Chapstick/lip balm
- ❑ Personal toiletries
- ❑ Nourishing clear liquids, 1-2 qts.
- ❑ Puddle pads
- ❑ Clothes to wear after the birth
- ❑ Fresh squeezed orange juice (for after the birth)

FOR COACH:
- ❑ Mother-to-be
- ❑ Quick Reference Guide
- ❑ Bradley® Coach Card
- ❑ Insurance Information for the Mom
- ❑ Copies of the Birth Plan

- ❑ Lotion for back rubs
- ❑ Tennis balls for back rubs
- ❑ Music & portable player w/fresh batteries, a/c cord
- ❑ Washcloths - at least 2
- ❑ Ice chest
- ❑ Flex straws
- ❑ Thermos of cold orange juice-at least two quarts
- ❑ Watch for timing contractions
- ❑ Personal toiletries
- ❑ Swim trunks
- ❑ Change of clothes
- ❑ Mobile phone/Phone card & Roll of coins (for calls)
- ❑ List of phone numbers
- ❑ Deck of cards or other games
- ❑ Food - snacks
- ❑ Party cups, plates, knife and napkins
- ❑ Camera, fresh film or memory and batteries
- ❑ Video and/or audio recorder
- ❑ Laptop computer for e-mail/pictures

FOR BABY:
NOTE: All clothes should be washed before use.
- ❑ Clothes to wear home
- ❑ Gown - undershirts
- ❑ Several receiving blankets
- ❑ 1 outer blanket
- ❑ Diapers (for newborn & babies 9+ lbs.)
- ❑ Pins (if cloth diapers)
- ❑ Baby book for footprints, etc.
- ❑ Birth-Day cake
- ❑ Puddle pad
- ❑ Blankets
- ❑ Infant car seat

Check with your birth team and include items they recommend.

©2010 AAHCC

STUDY HELPS

1. What information do you need to give informed consent?

2. List several ways the baby can be monitored. What are the advantages and disadvantages of each?

3. List several points made by Dr. Roberto Caldeyro-Barcia about normal labors.

4. What can the coach do to create a positive atmosphere in pregnancy, labor and birth?

5. What is the importance of emotional relaxation?

6. What is the normal length of gestation?

7. What value is there to natural pregnancy pre-labor (Braxton-Hicks) contractions? When do they most often begin, and what brings them on?

8. Write a brief description of your daily practice routine as you prepare for your labor and birth.

Class 1
Class 2
Class 3
Class 4
Class 5
Class 6
Class 7
Class 8
Class 9
Class 10
Class 11
Class 12

VARIATIONS AND UNEXPECTED SITUATIONS

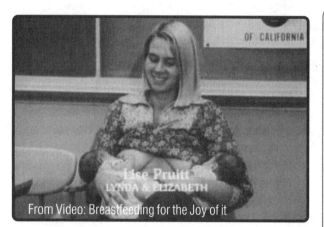

From Video: Breastfeeding for the Joy of it

Breech presentation: baby is coming foot, feet or buttocks first.

Cesarean section: surgical opening of abdomen and uterus to remove baby.

Due date: an educated guess as to the expected date of birth.

External version: turning the unborn baby by pressure through the mother's abdominal wall to alter the baby's position.

Meconium staining: appearance of bowel movement from baby in amniotic fluid prior to birth, a fairly common occurrence. Most often normal, but, rarely indicates distress.

Postmature baby: often merely means an error in estimating due date, or a pregnancy that really is longer than average. True postmaturity means, a seriously ill baby; placenta or mother not supplying needed nutrients, baby's skin is loose, baby losing weight, subcutaneous fat layer gone, baby looks like very old dying person. Very rare event.

Premature baby: a baby born before it is mature enough to thrive without assistance, not necessarily related to weight alone.

Full term: truly ready to be born, usually 40 to 43 weeks after conception.

Transverse lie: a baby lying sideways in the uterus, if the mother is in active labor this is a true complication. Very rare.

The vast majority of Bradley® couples will never need to use this information. In this class, we will spend some time discussing unusual situations and unpleasant possibilities. We cover this information so that you can feel confident in your ability to handle such a situation if it were to happen, however unlikely. Even if a complication arises and intervention becomes necessary, remember that it is still your baby's birth and can bring you joy.

As responsible parents, you must do whatever is necessary for the health and safety of mother and baby. Sometimes that means to stick with the natural process even when labor is a lot of hard work or more than you bargained for. Other times, that means choosing interventions and even a cesarean section, if that really becomes necessary. The attitude of the couple makes a difference. Look for the joy, and savor special moments under any circumstances.

GENERAL ASSIGNMENTS

❑ Nutrition and exercise as before.

❑ Walk: 20 min. 2X a day.

❑ Meet with birth team.

❑ Complete low risk worksheet - page 65.

❑ Relaxation practice: daily.

❑ Labor practice: daily.

❑ Pack your bags.

❑ Student Center: www.bradleybirth.com

❑ *Husband-Coached Childbirth*: chap. 15, 16.

❑ Fill out *Student Workbook*, pages 71-72.

EMOTIONAL RELAXATION

Emotional relaxation has to do with how you feel about what's happening to you in labor. It is especially important that the mother feel comfortable, so that her labor can progress normally. This week, work on emotional relaxation by paying special attention to the physical and verbal ways you protect and support your partner during relaxation practice. You should say a lot of things that are reassuring and calming to your partner. Protect and support her physically by keeping one hand on her body at all times and by sitting or standing in front of her to make her feel less vulnerable. Also set aside time to discuss feelings. Begin by just listening to each other's fears, thoughts, and anything she cares to express. Then work together on back-up plans, just in case any of these things happen. Finally, encourage her to let go of her fears and concentrate on the wonderful experience you are likely to have.

VARIATIONS

Definition	List some options:
Overdue: pregnancy continues beyond due date, an educated guess as to the date of birth.	- go to chiropractor - herbs - acupuncture
PROM: premature rupture of membranes.	
Herpes: herpes simplex type 2 lesions (sores) present in vaginal area of mother. May be life threatening if transmitted to baby. May be basis of recommendation of cesarean in cases of active lesions.	
OP: occiput posterior, baby's occipital bone (back of head) toward mother's back; "sunny-side-up". Causes "back labor".	- figure 8's - websters - inversion - pelvic rocking - acupuncture - labor in tub - sterile water injections in lower back
Breech: baby presenting foot, feet or buttocks first.	
Transverse: sideways: may be occiput transverse... where baby's occipital bone (back of head) is transverse, can temporarily occur when baby changes from posterior to anterior, and may not be a problem. Or may be a transverse lie... a baby presenting lying across the pelvic outlet which, in active labor, is a true obstetrical complication.	
Fast labor: labor shorter than average. (Average is about 15-17 hours.)	- shower/bath - side lying - relaxation - lay down horizontal - gravity neutral positions
Slow labor: labor longer than average.	- take stairs - walk - side lunge - ½ squat - change position - relaxation techniques - rest - eat & drink - make out
Reverse dilation: backward dilation, actually the closing rather than opening of the cervix. May be normal. May be error in measurement or the result of decreased pressure after the bag of waters breaks or perhaps the baby changing position. Usually progresses to previous dilation soon, without treatment.	

In class, it is only possible to discuss these things in generalities. Your particular case should be discussed in detail with your birth team. A certain unavoidable risk exists even with lots of preparation and the best medical support.

©2010 AAHCC

VARIATIONS

Class 1
Class 2
Class 3
Class 4
Class 5
Class 6
Class 7
Class 8
Class 9
Class 10
Class 11
Class 12

Definition	List some options:
Arrested labor: labor stops completely for a time, often is normal. Labor may resume soon, or days later.	– relaxation – stairs – change position – natural alignment plateau
Failure to progress: means failure to dilate fast enough. Overall progress, however, may be being achieved in other areas. Often given as a reason for a cesarean surgery. See: natural alignment plateau.	– stairs – walking – food intake – hydration – relaxation
Very painful labor: labor with above average levels of pain, may indicate a true problem.	– visualization – sterile water injection – vocalization – pelvic rocking – massaging – tens unit – tub
Meconium staining: common occurrence where amniotic fluid contains some meconium. Meconium is the baby's bowel movement. Most often normal, but rarely may indicate some distress. – proceed as normal – brown stain to amniotic fluid	– stairs – walking
CPD: cephalopelvic disproportion; baby's head bigger than pelvic outlet, while true CPD is extremely rare, CPD is often diagnosed and given as a cause for a cesarean surgery. True CPD can only be assessed after a generous amount of time in true second stage labor.	
Fetal distress: an unborn baby in trouble, often diagnosed by a fetal monitor, may be true distress, or a false reading or interpretation. Sometimes referred to as "Non-Reasuring Patterns".	
Multiple birth: twins, triplets and up.	

In class, it is only possible to discuss these things in generalities. Your particular case should be discussed in detail with your birth team. A certain unavoidable risk exists even with lots of preparation and the best medical support.

CESAREAN SURGERY

Attending classes and preparing for a joyous, natural, Bradley® birth is the best preparation for any unusual situation that may arise. As you learn in class, most couples experience the type of birth they have their hearts set on. Once in a while, a well-trained couple needs to have a cesarean section for a valid medical reason. These couples should be just as proud of themselves as other couples, since they worked just as hard (perhaps harder) and did the best they could for their baby. Babies born to couples who attend Bradley® classes generally do better than other cesarean babies, because they often have medication only minutes or seconds before the surgical birth. Although the contractions of the uterus may not have led to a vaginal birth, they are important in massaging and preparing your baby for life. Note that many unprepared vaginal births are medicated for hours before birth. Your baby may actually have received less narcotics than many vaginally-born babies.

DOING YOUR BEST TO KEEP A CESAREAN FROM BECOMING NECESSARY

Some indications for cesarean are beyond your control, and medical technology could save you or your baby's life. However, a cesarean can become necessary because of poor earlier choices (inadequate nutrition, use of drugs, lack of exercise, etc.) or lack of preparation.

1. Do everything you can to keep yourself healthy and low risk.

2. Be committed to having a natural birth. Remember that there are potentially dangerous side effects to every drug and procedure. The risk to the mother's and baby's lives may be multiplied many times by cesarean section.

3. Have a well-trained coach.

4. Understand and work with the natural process. (See B.E.S.T. techniques.)

5. Choose your birth place and birth team wisely and have good communications with them.

A DIFFICULT DECISION
(for the parents and their doctor)

1. Listen to your doctor's explanation of the situation.

2. Discuss any alternatives. Weigh the benefits against the risks. (See questions for informed consent on Positive Communications page.)

3. Express your feelings.

4. Ask for some time together to calm down, make your decision, and adjust to this new situation.

5. Call your Bradley® instructor for support.

Class 1 Class 2 Class 3 Class 4 Class 5 Class 6 Class 7 Class 8 Class 9 Class 10 Class 11 Class 12

WHEN A CESAREAN IS NECESSARY ...

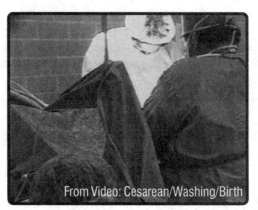

From Video: Cesarean/Washing/Birth

How to handle it

1. Communicate. Ask the surgical team to help explain, step-by-step, what is about to happen.

2. Surgery requires many compromises, but many choices may still be available.

CHOICES CHECKLIST

- ❏ Coach present
- ❏ Mother awake during surgery
- ❏ Ether screen lowered so mom can see baby No'
- ❏ Immediate photographs
- ❏ Mother having contact with baby soon after birth
- ❏ Mother having one hand free to touch baby
- ❏ Breastfeeding soon
- ❏ Gentle handling of baby (if possible)

- ❏ Coach holding baby in operating room
- ❏ Oxygen mask removed so mother can talk to baby
- ❏ Family bonding period after the surgery
- ❏ Family/father stay with baby if going to nursery
- ❏ Minimal nursery stay
- ❏ Delayed or no bathing (to avoid temperature drop, separation)
- ❏ Parental consent for newborn procedures
- ❏ Rooming-in

3. A pediatrician must be present because of the increased risk for the baby. Will your pediatrician attend, or will you need to use one on staff at the hospital?

4. Make the best of it and have a good experience. This is your baby's birth. Your relaxation techniques will still be very useful.

THINGS TO REMEMBER

Remember this is the birth of your baby no matter how it is born. There are special things you should remember and tell your Bradley® teacher about.
1. What did the baby look like the first time you saw him/her?
2. What was the baby's color... pink from the start? Bluish? How soon did it pink up?
3. What did the baby's eyes look like... alert, sleepy? Did you look into your baby's eyes?
4. What did the baby feel like the first time you touched him/her?
5. What did the baby smell like? There is a newborn smell!
6. Did the baby have hair? What color? Wet or dry? Short or long?
7. How soon did the baby respond to your touch or voice?

Take pictures and write your responses down. Ask the mother the same things. This is what you want to remember; the baby & the joy of birth.

Class 1
Class 2
Class 3
Class 4
Class 5
Class 6
Class 7
Class 8
Class 9
Class 10
Class 11
Class 12

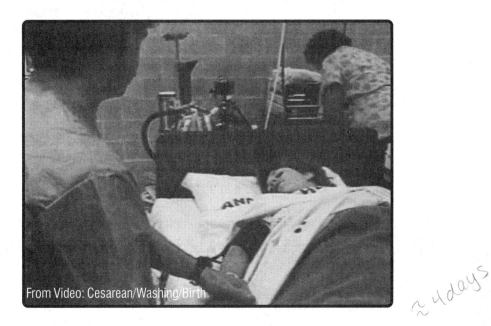

RECOVERING FROM A CESAREAN

From Video: Cesarean/Washing/Birth

≈4days

These are some suggestions from other mothers. They may or may not apply in your case.

1. Early ambulation (12-14 hours after surgery). Stand tall and walk slowly, making sure you lift your feet as you walk.

2. Use a pillow to support incision when coughing, sneezing, or holding baby.

3. Minimize gas by eating lightly soon after delivery (ask doctor to leave an order for light nourishment), walking, avoiding hot or iced fluids, eating roughage, whole grain cereals and breads. Don't use drinking straws.

4. Spinal headaches may be helped by drinking lots of fluids and lying flat.

5. If allowed, abdominal tightening may begin immediately in recovery room. It may lessen or eliminate gas pains. Take a breath and exhale, then inhale and hold for a count of five; finally, exhale slowly. Do three times every hour (periodically) for 5 days.

6. Contact La Leche League for help with breastfeeding after surgery. Cesarean babies may need your colostrum and breastmilk even more than those born vaginally.

7. Contact a cesarean support group in your area. After a surgical birth, parents may need to talk.

8. Remember to ask your doctor about VBAC next time. Many doctors are now doing vaginal births after cesareans.

9. Call your Bradley® instructor. Please return your follow-up form and bring your baby back to class. We care about you. We want to see you and your baby and hear your story.

Class 1 | Class 2 | Class 3 | Class 4 | Class 5 | Class 6 | Class 7 | **Class 8** | Class 9 | Class 10 | Class 11 | Class 12

COMPLICATIONS

Evaluate each situation as it arises.

Ask: Is the mother okay?
Is the baby okay?
What is the problem?

Consider: Can this be normal?
What are we afraid might happen?
How much time do we have?
What choices do we have?

Remember to think about all three of you.
Ask for explanations so that you can understand if and why intervention might be necessary.

1. If a complication arises during active labor, she will rely on you to act as an advocate for her. Are you aware of all her feelings regarding the "what if" situations?

2. What are you most afraid could happen?

3. If that did happen, what could you do to handle it in a positive way?

4. Though the situations listed below may not be a part of the natural childbirth you're planning, they do, on occasion, become necessary because of complications. For the situations that could possibly apply to you, describe what you could do to handle each of them in a positive way if they were to occur.

   Premature rupture of membranes (PROM):

   A need for an I.V.:

   A need to use an internal fetal monitor:

   Being transferred from homebirth or out-of-hospital birth center to hospital:

   A suggestion to induce or augment labor:

   If the fetal monitor indicates distress:

   The need for a cesarean surgery:

5. What can be some normal reasons for backward dilation of the cervix?

6. What changes need to be made if there is a lip or rim of cervix?

7. Is it possible for a first time mother to deliver a posterior baby vaginally?

8. Is meconium staining always a sign of distress?

• *Most labors and births are normal.*

• *Good communications with your birth team will enhance your experience.*

• *There are no absolute guarantees that everything will go well.*

• *Because the mother has done what she could to stay healthy and low risk, she and the baby are more likely to handle a complication better.*

• *Each labor is unique. Only the mother and coach can make the important decisions that will have to be made in labor.*

• *No matter what happens, you can call your Bradley® instructor for support.*

Class 1
Class 2
Class 3
Class 4
Class 5
Class 6
Class 7
Class 8
Class 9
Class 10
Class 11
Class 12

ARE YOU DOING EVERYTHING YOU CAN TO STAY HEALTHY AND LOW RISK?

I. NUTRITION - Each day, are you getting a well-balanced diet including:

Yes No   *How could you improve?*

- ❑ ❑ 80-100 grams of complete protein? _____
  (try to include: 2 protein servings, 4 servings milk, 2 servings eggs)
- ❑ ❑ 2 servings of dark green, leafy vegetables? _____
- ❑ ❑ 4 or more servings bread, rice, tortilla, potato, etc.? _____
- ❑ ❑ 1 or 2 vitamin C foods? _____
- ❑ ❑ 3 servings of fats? _____
- ❑ ❑ 1 serving fruit other than citrus? _____
- ❑ ❑ 1 serving of another vegetable? _____
- ❑ ❑ 1 serving whole grain cereal? _____
- ❑ ❑ Adequate fluids, 8-10 glasses water, juice, etc. (drink to thirst)? _____
- ❑ ❑ Adequate salt (salt to taste)? _____

II. EXERCISE - If your physical condition permits, each day are you striving to do:

- ❑ ❑ Some form of physical exercise (10-20 minutes, twice)? _____
- ❑ ❑ Plenty of tailor sitting? _____
- ❑ ❑ Plenty of squats? _____
- ❑ ❑ 40 pelvic rocks 4 times daily & 80 before bed? _____
- ❑ ❑ 10 butterfly exercises? _____
- ❑ ❑ 200 Kegels? _____

III. EDUCATION - Have you:

- ❑ ❑ Been attending classes regularly? _____
- ❑ ❑ Finished reading *Husband-Coached Childbirth*? _____
- ❑ ❑ Read *Children At Birth*? _____
- ❑ ❑ Read *Womanly Art of Breastfeeding*? _____
- ❑ ❑ Read *Natural Childbirth the Bradley® Way*? _____

Class 1 Class 2 Class 3 Class 4 Class 5 Class 6 Class 7 **Class 8** Class 9 Class 10 Class 11 Class 12

❏ ❏ Completed the breastfeeding questionnaire? _____

❏ ❏ Completed your birth plan? _____

❏ ❏ Felt a need to learn more about any particular subject? _____

IV. AVOIDANCE OF THINGS THAT MAY BE HARMFUL: Are you being careful to avoid:

❏ ❏ Drugs of all kinds? _____

❏ ❏ Exposure to cigarette smoke? _____

❏ ❏ Alcohol? _____

❏ ❏ Artificial sweeteners (aspartame, NutraSweet®, etc.)? _____

❏ ❏ Mercury and aluminum? _____

❏ ❏ Chemicals (including household types)? _____

❏ ❏ Pesticides? _____

❏ ❏ Caffeine? _____

❏ ❏ Additives and preservatives? _____

❏ ❏ Junk foods (white flour, sugar, chocolate, etc.)? _____

❏ ❏ Vaginal exams, unless absolutely necessary? _____

❏ ❏ Ultrasound exposure and interventions, unless absolutely necessary? _____
(including doptone)

V. RELAXATION - Each day are you:

❏ ❏ Practicing relaxation twice (at least once with your coach)? _____

❏ ❏ Getting the kind of support from your coach that you need? _____

❏ ❏ Getting adequate rest, even if that requires taking a nap? _____

❏ ❏ Careful to avoid excessive stress? _____

❏ ❏ Content with the plans you have made for this birth? _____

❏ ❏ Careful not to overdo it at home or at work? _____

❏ ❏ Able to set aside a few minutes to do something you really enjoy? _____

❏ ❏ Sure that your coach is adequately rested, in case labor begins soon? _____

Left margin tabs: Class 1, Class 2, Class 3, Class 4, Class 5, Class 6, Class 7, **Class 8**, Class 9, Class 10, Class 11, Class 12

POSTPARTUM PREPARATION

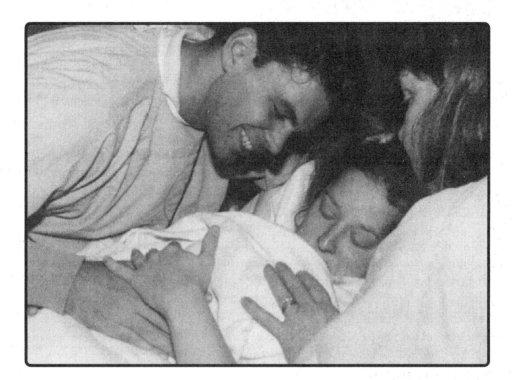

So much time is devoted to getting ready for the birth that many couples forget how important it is to prepare in advance for the first few weeks following the birth. It is a time of great change, physically, mentally, emotionally, and within the family. Things will never be the same. The baby will enrich your life.

Everybody is different. Some women regain their energy faster than others. These are suggestions other women have tried and found successful. You will have to find what works best for you. If you have any problems that cannot be resolved, get help from your doctor, Bradley® instructor, La Leche League leader or others in your community willing to help.

VOCABULARY

Afterbirth pains: additional contractions of the uterus after the birth is completed which help return the uterus to it's proper size, and reduce blood loss.

typically during breastfeeding - lasts a week or 2

Areola: the darkened ring surrounding the nipple of the breast.

Colostrum: "nature's vaccine for the newborn" (AAP), fluid in breast prior to the milk "coming in".

Involution: return of the uterus to it's normal size and position after birth.

Lactation: breastfeeding; the function of secreting milk.

LLL: La Leche League; a group of experienced mothers who help support good mothering through breastfeeding.

Lochia: the bloody discharge for several weeks following birth. *bleed 3-6 weeks after birth*

Pediatrician: a practitioner of the branch of medicine dealing with children.

Postpartum: the period after a baby is born.

Recovery: often used to describe the immediate period after a birth, surgery or procedure.

TAKING CARE OF YOURSELF - POSTPARTUM

The following are suggestions from thousands of mothers. Your doctor may have additional suggestions or changes specific to your case.

SUGGESTED SUPPLIES

3-6 Nursing bras
2-4 Gowns
2-4 Light robes
2 Boxes hospital size or overnight sanitary pads
1-2 Boxes maxi pads
Nursing/postpartum clothes (between pregnant and non-pregnant size)
Puddle pads
Something to put ice in, or blue ice with a cover
Snacks
Drinks (100% juice, water, milk)
Large glass and pitcher
Easy to prepare meals and ready snacks

RIGHT AFTER THE BABY IS BORN

Your first thought is one of delight, perhaps surprise, and thanks... that the hard work of labor is over. You may also experience feelings of loss or baby blues at the same time. This is normal and generally passes quickly. You need some rest and some good food now.

Bonding

A normal baby should be able to stay with the mother continuously so the family can bond and nursing can get off to a great start.

Getting Acquainted With Your New Baby

Human mothers have a "sensitive period" immediately after delivery. Dr. Klaus found that human mothers who were allowed contact with their babies in this sensitive period were more responsive to their infants' needs, were reluctant to leave them in the care of others, showed greater sensitivity to the infants' cries and made greater efforts to soothe them.

Episiotomy and Stitches

If you had an episiotomy, the doctor may give you a local for the stitches after the cord has been cut, thus the drugs do not transfer to the baby's circulation. Intermittant ice packs are generally recommended for the first 24 hours to reduce swelling. Taking warm sitz baths frequently after that usually feels good. Doing Kegel exercises may also be helpful.

Nursing

Immediately after the baby is born is a critical learning period. Proper nursing position assists the mother to avoid severe problems with engorgement and sore nipples.

1. Mother should be sitting up or on her side.
2. Hold baby's head in crook of arm with hand cradling bottom.
3. Turn baby tummy to tummy with mother.
4. Only mother should touch baby while getting baby on breast. Baby's head is sensitive and will turn to touch.
5. Tickle baby's cheek with nipple.
6. Wait until baby opens mouth and tongue is down.
7. Guide breast into babies mouth with other hand (C shape, cupped under breast with thumb on top).
8. Pull baby close, using cradling arm.

Most babies will nurse for 5-10 minutes or longer on one side and then as long as they want on the other side. For the next feeding, start on the other side. Often they fall asleep at the breast. If you need to take the baby off the breast, slide your finger between the breast and the corner of the baby's mouth to break the suction. Never pull the baby off the breast. You may feel like you are nursing all the time, this is normal. Some newborns nurse as often as every twenty minutes in the beginning, others nurse only every one or two hours.

Shaking

You may experience a shaky, chilly sensation which is due to physiological changes. Shaking may last for 1-2 hours.

Massage

The nurse will show you how to massage the uterus to help involution.

Iced Orange Juice

Tastes good and is important to help restore depleted blood sugar, potassium and fluids.

Walking

Walking soon after birth helps to restore circulation and expel blood clots. Be sure you have a normal birth, drink orange juice, have breastfed the baby, and feel good before walking.

Urinating for the First Time

You may not realize you need to urinate and may have trouble figuring out how because of swelling. Relax, listen to the sound of running water, pour water over yourself. Only very rarely is it necessary to catheterize for urinary retention.

Soreness

You may have sore muscles you never knew you had. Remember, warm baths, rest, and massage can help. This was an athletic event.

AT HOME

The average hospital stay for natural Bradley® trained childbirth patients is 2 to 24 hours. Certain conditions should be met before going home early:

1. Natural birth (unmedicated).
2. Normal recovery.
3. Breastfeeding well.
4. Help at home. (Husband?)
5. Knowledge of what is normal for yourself and your new baby.
6. Healthy mother, healthy baby.

Rest, Rest, Rest

This is the most important thing you need. Get help with the housework, dishes, shopping, etc. You are capable of taking care of yourself and the baby, nothing else.

Lying on Your Stomach

Place a pillow on the bed and lie on your stomach a few minutes each day. This helps the uterus to contract, expel blood clots and get back to its normal size.

Visitors

Keep visits short. If guests ask to help, tell them how. Wear your bathrobe when guests arrive, they won't stay as long.

Engorgement

Sometimes the breasts become hard and swollen when the milk first comes in (this may be prevented by nursing frequently). It may be necessary to soften the breast by taking a shower or forming the nipple with your hand. Engorgement goes away quickly.

Breast Care

Regular bathing is important, but be careful to avoid getting soap on your nipples. Wearing a nursing bra for support will help heavy breasts. Change bras frequently as they get wet.

Leaking

At home, sometimes it feels best to just let the breast leak into a clean diaper. If you are out, you may want to put padding into your bra such as a folded cloth or handkerchief. Plastic-lined breast shields may lead to a breast infection. Placing the heel of your hand against the nipple or folding your arms against the breast may stop the leaking.

Sore Nipples

Be sure the baby latches on correctly. Try nursing in other positions, or put the baby in another position, such as the football hold. If this becomes a problem call your local La Leche League leader.

Breast Infections

A breast infection is indicated by a hot, sore breast or spot, possibly with a fever. Rest, heat pad, and frequent nursing generally help. Call your doctor, if it persists. Often this is caused by overdoing it.

Diet

Keep on a good diet full of protein, fluids, fruits and vegetables. Continue the same vitamin-iron supplement as prescribed during pregnancy, at least until the doctor or birth attendant checks you.

Emotions

You usually feel very elated, unless you do not get enough rest or don't have good enough nutrition. Then, "after baby blues" may occur.

Lochia

Bloody discharge following birth lasting up to 6 weeks. You should notice a significant decrease after 4 days. It begins bright red, then changes to a light pink or brown color. Saturating 2 pads (hospital size) within 1 hour is too much. Call your doctor. Once the flow has changed, a bright red color and increased amount generally indicates you are overdoing it. Rest. If rest does not help, call your doctor.

Class 1
Class 2
Class 3
Class 4
Class 5
Class 6
Class 7
Class 8
Class 9
Class 10
Class 11
Class 12

First Bowel Movement

In order to make this comfortable, avoid constipation by drinking plenty of fluids, eating fruit and high-fiber foods. Do Kegels, and put feet on a stool when going to the bathroom (this simulates squatting position).

Hemorrhoids

These sometimes occur. Many women find getting off their feet, taking hot baths, and doing Kegels help. If they persist, check with your doctor.

Lovemaking

OK, after you are checked by your doctor. The first time may be very tender; take it easy. Dr. Bradley recommended using K-Y jelly to help lubrication, which may be lacking during lactation.

Afterbirth "Pains"

These are contractions of the uterus, just as before birth. Use relaxation and abdominal breathing. Your uterus is contracting back to normal.

Exercises After the Birth

Kegel - with your doctor's OK. Begin right after birth and continue daily. They should be done for life.

Pelvic Rock - Begin as soon as your doctor says. (Usually when the lochial flow subsides.) This exercise is great for afterbirth "pains," backache, and strengthening abdominal muscles. It is actually better than sit ups and leg lifts, which may not be good for you. The pelvic rock is another "lifetime" exercise. Exercises for True Natural Childbirth by Rhondda Hartman, RN, AAHCC.

Exercises After Your Check Up

Continue with Kegel, pelvic rock, tailor sitting.

Lie on back with knees raised. Raise back and head as you reach for left knee with right hand. Relax. Do other side. Repeat, twice.

In standing position, take abdominal breath, let air out. Now expel residual air and hold. (Feel abdominal muscles tighten.) Inhale; relax. Repeat twice each day.

Regular exercise is, perhaps, more likely to be continued if, after six weeks, you take up some kind of sport you like. Start slowly and remember to tune-in to your body.

Exercises to Avoid

Do not do sit ups, leg lifts, complete knee bends.

check with healthcare professional before beginning exercise program.

Take it easy

Remember, you have just had a baby. Do not overdo exercising. Take it slowly to begin with, and increase activity gradually. Get plenty of rest, sleep when baby sleeps, and do not try to assume responsibility for the complete household. Eat plenty of nutritious food and drink ample fluids. Enjoy your baby.

On Being a Family

Other members of your family need to be included in this exciting event. Grandparents, other relatives, friends, and especially your other children might enjoy being present at the birth. If your other small children were not at the birth, they might enjoy sitting in the middle of the bed to hold the new baby. Daddy can hold the baby skin-to-skin by taking off his shirt. Babies love to hear Daddy's heartbeat and snuggle up to his body.

DANGER SIGNS

Bleeding - Saturating two large pads in less than an hour.

Breast pain - Sudden pain or continued pain when nursing; redness and unusual swelling.

Fever - Elevated temperature (over 100.4F).

Dizziness or fainting - Persistent or repetitive spells of light-headedness.

Episiotomy pain - Sudden onset of new pain or swelling at the site of the episiotomy.

Infection - Any of the classical signs of infection, particularly foul-smelling lochia (discharge), elevated temperature, unusual pain in abdomen, swelling of the vagina, rapid pulse.

Pain - Any sharp or unexpected pain.

Depression - Severe.

Urination problems - Urinating just a teaspoon at a time or with pain or difficulty.

Don't spend time or energy worrying. If you are concerned, call your doctor.

From The Birth Center, by Salee Berman, CNM and Victor Berman, MD.

POSTPARTUM CARE

HOUSEWORK

After the baby is born, the mother will need time to recover. She should be able to take care of herself and her baby, and that is all. Over-activity may lead to increased bleeding which causes exhaustion, loss of weight too fast and loss of breast milk. Someone else will need to handle the housework and other responsibilities for at least the first two weeks. After the baby is two weeks old, the mother can probably begin doing some of the smaller chores around the house, but will need continued assistance until the first six weeks have passed. Eventually, she and the baby will settle into some normal patterns. But be aware that this will not be like getting back to normal, it will be more like finding a new norm.

This worksheet was designed to help the mother and her assistant, or assistants, prepare for this time. We recommend that you do everything you can ahead of time to make things as easy as possible for everyone. We also suggest that you set up a practice day when everyone actually performs their assigned tasks. Remember to fill in the worksheet completely, and HAVE FUN!

"CAN I DO SOMETHING TO HELP?"

List ways that willing friends and neighbors could help you:_____

_____

_____

_____

_____

Who will be responsible for these jobs?

❏ Laundry :_____.

❏ Dishes :_____.

❏ Shopping :_____.

❏ Cooking :_____.

❏ Cleaning :_____.

Notes and special instructions:_____

_____

_____

_____

_____

Class 1 Class 2 Class 3 Class 4 Class 5 Class 6 Class 7 Class 8 Class 9 Class 10 Class 11 Class 12

Class 1 | Class 2 | Class 3 | Class 4 | Class 5 | Class 6 | Class 7 | **Class 8** | Class 9 | Class 10 | Class 11 | Class 12

DAILY CHORES

Carefully consider your priorities. What chores really must be done every day? What can you let go for a while? List the jobs that really need to be done in order of importance.

What needs to be done?	Who will do it?	Notes:
_____	_____	_____
_____	_____	_____
_____	_____	_____
_____	_____	_____

WEEKLY CHORES

What needs to be done?	Who will do it?	Notes:
_____	_____	_____
_____	_____	_____
_____	_____	_____

IF YOU HAVE OTHER CHILDREN

Have you been educating them on pregnancy, birth and newborns?

Who will help you take care of them?

What are their normal schedules?
    Morning-

    Afternoon-

    Evening-

What will you do to make them feel special and important?

What will you do to involve them in caring for the baby?

What things are fun for them to do at home?

Where could they go for a special outing?

ADVANCED FIRST STAGE TECHNIQUES

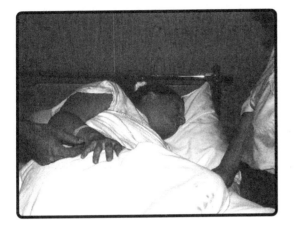

Mucous plug: a blob of mucous passed by the mother as the cervix begins to dilate. May be well before the onset of labor.
Multigravida: a woman who has been pregnant two or more times.
Multipara: a woman who has given birth to two or more babies.
Parturition: the act of birthing.
Positive pain: pain with a purpose, whose meaning is to inform you of progress, needed changes, etc..
Pre-labor: before labor.
Primigravida: a woman during her first pregnancy.
Supine position: lying on your back.
Vaginal exam: entering the vagina usually with gloved fingers to assess the dilation, effacement, descent, position, etc. May increase the risk of infection.

You can learn how to work with your body to shorten labor, reduce pain and make your experience more enjoyable. When you know how to do something right, it is almost always easier.

We cover a lot of different variables and teach a variety of techniques because you and your labor are one of a kind. The natural process is well-designed and accommodates many variations.

RAINBOW

This technique deals with mental relaxation and can be done in any position. If you have not yet experimented with various positions this would be a good time to start. Begin your daily relaxation practice periods this week by getting your partner physically relaxed. Once you feel she is physically relaxed, begin this guided imagery. "Allow yourself to imagine as though you had a large movie screen just in front of your eyes and you are able to project onto that screen the color red. Imagine an object that is a very deep red. A deep red image firmly in your mind." (pause) "Now allow that image to change to orange, as you picture a bright orange object on the movie screen before you." Continue through the colors of the rainbow (red to orange, to yellow, to green, to blue, to violet, then to white and bright white). Pause between each color and observe the changes as her mind and body relax.

GENERAL ASSIGNMENTS

☐ *Husband-Coached Childbirth*: Chap. 17-20.

☐ Relaxation practice daily.

☐ Continue nutrition and exercise.

☐ Walk 25 min and 20 min a day.

☐ Student Center: www.bradleybirth.com

©2010 AAHCC

WORKING WITH YOUR BODY
Study Guide

PREPARATION FOR LABOR

1. What can the mother do during pregnancy to stay healthy and low risk?

2. What things should be done before the labor begins so that the mother avoids any unnecessary pain in labor?

3. What should the mother and coach be doing for at least twenty minutes each day so that they will be best able to handle any pain in labor?

4. How are due dates determined and how accurate are they?

5. What do contractions feel like?

TYPICAL CHARACTERISTICS

1. What are the typical physical and emotional signs during each of these.

PRE-LABOR	EARLY FIRST STAGE	LATE FIRST STAGE	N.A.P.
Generally: • Contractions are irregular. • They last less than 60 seconds. • May contract on side, top, bottom, all over. • May subside from changing activity or eating. • Mom is excited, active, hungry, thirsty, still modest.	Generally: • Contractions are 10 minutes apart or less. • They last 45- 60 seconds. • So strong Mom stops and concentrates for contractions. • Will not space out from activity change. • Adrenalin still has an effect. • Contractions become progessively stronger and closer together. • Acceptance, "This is it!"	Generally: • Contractions are quite close together. • They last 60 seconds or more. • Contractions are *extremely* intense. • She is no longer hungry. • She is loosing her modesty. • There is no doubt she is in labor. • Mother has serious behavior, "Do Not Disturb" attitude.	Generally: • Contractions continue to come close together. • They continue to be extremely intense. • All signs are same as late first stage except... • No increase in dilation. • May need time to: align, increase size of pelvis, prepare colostrum, prep. baby for breathing, etc.. • May end in rapid complete dilation.

PRE-LABOR (Braxton-Hicks Contractions)

1. *If you are unsure this is labor Dr. Bradley said try to:*

•*Eat*   •*Drink*   •*Walk*   •*Shower*   •*Nap*

2. How do you coach a woman in pre-labor?

3. Why do some parents go to the hospital once or twice before their actual labor?

4. Why is pre-labor important?

FIRST STAGE LABOR

1. What positions would be good for the mother to assume during early first stage?

2. What position would not be good for the mother to assume during first stage or anytime during pregnancy?

3. What position opens the inlet of the pelvis to help the baby come down?

4. What position is most likely to speed the labor?

5. What position is least likely to speed the labor?

6. If you are going to change locations during labor, what things can you do to make the move less stressful?

7. What prepping procedures are standard for your place of birth?

8. What can you do to make your birth center or hospital more home-like?

9. Under what conditions should you consider going home and returning later to the hospital?
   - less than 5cm dialated, not showing signs of late labor

10. What can the coach do to create a positive environment and attitude at the hospital, birth center, or at home?

11. What can be done during labor to avoid unnecessary pain:

PHYSICALLY	MENTALLY	EMOTIONALLY
Work with, not against your body. • Urinate often. • Don't lie on back. • Freedom to move about. • Drink. • Eat. • etc.	Being in a relaxed environment. Hearing or thinking relaxing thoughts and or sounds. • Music. • Stories. • Poems. • Dim lights. • Comfortable temperature.	Emotional support of coach. • Reassurance. • Praise. • Confidence. • Positive Communications.

12. How can the mother best handle hard labor contractions and any pain she does experience?

13. What are the seven things on the coach's check list?

Class 1
Class 2
Class 3
Class 4
Class 5
Class 6
Class 7
Class 8
Class 9
Class 10
Class 11
Class 12

14. What techniques can be used by the coach to encourage physical relaxation?

15. What can the coach do to encourage mental relaxation?

16. What can the coach do to encourage emotional relaxation?

17. What are the different sensations the mother might be feeling in late first stage labor?

18. What might a mother in this stage be thinking, but be unable to say?

NATURAL ALIGNMENT PLATEAU

1. What are the four things measured during a vaginal exam?

2. What other things are happening in the mother which need to be completed before the baby should be born?

3. What things are happening in the baby which need to be completed before the baby is ready to be born?

4. What can a coach do for a mother who is experiencing a "Natural Alignment Plateau" (N.A.P.)?

5. List positive, relaxing phrases that you could use in labor:

JUDGING THE PROGRESS OF LABOR

1. What signs could help you to recognize each stage of labor?

	Emotional/Behavioral	Contractions	Mother's Description	Clothing
Early First Stage	Excitement/acceptance "Putsy-putsy"	10 minutes apart or less 45-60 seconds long	"Wow, these are strong contractions"	Modest
Active First Stage	Seriousness "Do Not Disturb"	Quite close together 60 seconds or more	"Shh"	Less Modest
Transition	Self doubt Confession "I give up"	One on top of each other Double peak, space out, stop	"I dont think I can do this anymore!"	Little Modesty
Second Stage	Calmness & Determination	Space out again approximately 60 seconds long	"Here it comes again honey... breath"	No Modesty

2. Remember, the average length of first stage labor is 15-17 hours. Varies from a few hours to a few days.

3. Five centimeters dilated? Could be: pre-labor, 1st stage, transition, or entering 2nd stage.

4. What signs might help you to determine whether you are having an average or slow labor (and should stay calm and conserve your energy) or a fast labor (and should quickly prepare for the birth)?

Possible signs of slow labor	Possible signs of average labor	Possible signs of fast labor
Contractions start and stop. 10-20 minutes apart. Extremely variable. Not getting closer, longer, or stronger.	Fairly regular contractions: 10 minutes or less. 60 seconds or longer. Becoming closer, longer, and stronger by the hour.	Contractions begin close, long, and extremely strong. Active labor signs from beginning.

5. If you are not sure this is the real thing, Dr. Bradley says to try 5 things:

    1. ☐ Eat   2. ☐ Drink   3. ☐ Walk   4. ☐ Shower   5. ☐ Nap

6. Still unsure? Try the above again.

7. Most labors follow a pattern. Some labors start & stop.

8. How would you handle the challenge of the following situation? For a few hours, you are in active labor, and then it stops. Hours or days later, it starts up, only to stop again. (This can be a normal variation.) In any case conserve your energy! Rest when you can, eat & drink as normal.

• *There is no accurate way to determine when labor will begin.*

• *There is no accurate way to predict how long the labor will take or what challenges you will face during that time.*

• *It is challenging to decide when to leave for your birth place or to call in your birth team. Couples are understandably nervous and are much more likely to do this way too early than too late.*

• *Some labors progress very quickly and then may seem to stall for many hours and vice versa. The natural alignment plateau occurs in over 30% of natural labors.*

• *The idea that dilation of the cervix, timing of contractions, or any other measurement will tell you where you are in labor is a myth. Averages exist, but you are not an average. Piece together all of your information to get an idea of what's happening.*

Class 1 Class 2 Class 3 Class 4 Class 5 Class 6 Class 7 Class 8 **Class 9** Class 10 Class 11 Class 12

Class 1
Class 2
Class 3
Class 4
Class 5
Class 6
Class 7
Class 8
Class 9
Class 10
Class 11
Class 12

ASSISTING A LABORING WOMAN

1. Part of The Bradley® philosophy is to "tune-in to your body." As the coach, you need to take your cues from the mother and to encourage her to do what she feels like doing. Women in labor are sometimes confused; this technique will help her to make decisions.

Give an example using this technique:

A. Ask her. "What would you like to do now, and how can I help you?"
    If she doesn't know, then ...

A. Ask her:

B. List the choices. "Which of these would you like to do, and how can I help you?"
    If she can't decide . . .

B. List the choices:

C. Suggest to her. "We are going to try this and see what you think." (If she does not want to try that, choose another option.)

C. Suggest to her:

2. Refer to list of ways that you and your partner have handled discomfort, pain and stress in your lives from class 1.

3. Remember things you can do to help your partner avoid unnecessary pain in labor.

4. What are your partner's favorite ways of handling pain?

5. Types of pain may relate to progress in labor. The lower the pressure the lower the baby; the stronger the contraction, the sooner the birth.

6. Explain why the technique of relating pain with progress can be helpful.

7. What can you give your partner other than medication, if she says, "Give me something for the pain!"
   • *a hug*   • *a compliment*   • *an encouraging phrase*   • *a rub*   • *attention*

8. How can you avoid being separated in these situations?
   • *Parking car* • *Fast labor* • *Exam* • *Mom in bathroom* • *Admitting*   • *Prepping* • *Cesarean* • *Shower*

9. Ways you can assist your partner if she has a backache.
   • *Upper back rub* • *Lower rub* • *Fist low* • *Hip squeeze* • *Massage shoulders* • *Lower pressure* • *Heel upward*

10. Places you can massage her if she doesn't want her torso touched.
    • *Hair* • *Temples* • *Feet* • *Legs* • *Arms* • *Neck* • *Hands*

11. Things you can say and talk about if she needs constant verbal coaching.
    • *A place you have been* • *Rainbow* • *Baby* • *Future* • *etc.*

___

• *Every labor is different. You will not know what works best for you until you are in labor.*

• *In labor, you may have a better idea of how well she's doing than she does.*

• *Giving birth is a lot of hard work and can be painful. She is counting on you to help her avoid unnecessary pain and handle the pain that's left over by using relaxation techniques you've learned.*

• *Often medication does not eliminate the pain.*

• *Remember the Hawthorne effect: your just being there makes a tremendous difference.*

COMMUNICATING WITH YOUR BIRTH TEAM

1. Write out an example of what you might say when you first meet with your birth team during labor. Set up a positive attitude, brief them on what's happened to that point, remind them of your special desires for this birth (keep it to a few of the most important points), and suggest to them some ways that they can help you.

2. What possible situation are you the most worried about? Explain how, if it did happen, you would handle it in a positive way that is most likely to get the result you desire?

3. How will the way you are dressed affect the way you are treated?

4. Give an example of how you would use the following technique to encourage a friendly attitude:
   A. Use first names:

   B. Give honest appreciation: "Thank you for... ."

   C. Suggest ways they can assist you: "Please, can you help us by... ?"

• *Your birth team is concerned with your health and safety.*

• *They are trained in the management of abnormality and can assist you in case of complications.*

• *You may need to suggest ways that they can help you during a normal labor.*

• *The birth team is made up of people. Be considerate of their feelings.*

• *Your positive example will help others, especially if your birth team is not familiar with The Bradley Method®.*

• *Show your coach card to your birth team so they will know you are well-trained.*

CLASS 10 (week 10 of 12)
ADVANCED SECOND STAGE TECHNIQUES

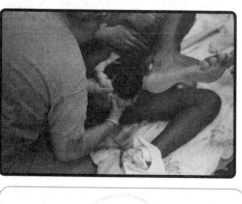

Crowning: the portion of second stage labor when the baby's head pushes the tissues forward looking like a crown.

Local anesthetic: an injection of a narcotic in the skin, which will soon spread to the whole body and the baby. "There is no such thing as a local." (Dr. Bradley).

Perineal massage: massaging lotion on the perineum. Purpose: to thin the perineum and add to it's elasticity... may reduce chance of tearing or need for episiotomy.

Placenta: the afterbirth; organ grown from outer layer of the egg which grows to nourish the baby... mother's blood and baby's blood circulate and transfer oxygen, nutrients, wastes... but do not mix.

Posterior presentation: baby's occipital bone (back of head) is facing mothers back. Causes "back labor".

Pressure episiotomy: PE; episiotomy performed without narcotics, birth attendant waits until crowning, cuts during a contraction when the stretched perineum is without circulation and sensation is naturally reduced.

Sitz baths: warm, shallow water bath.

Third stage: expulsion of the placenta.

Umbilical cord: connects the baby to it's placenta. Contains two arteries and one vein. Is also a part of endocrine system, manufactures hormones.

Presentation (Vertex or Breech): vertex is the top of the head, breech is either buttocks, foot or feet first.

Labor changes now. Often there are longer rest periods. Relaxing with contractions is for first stage. Active participation is what is needed now. Second stage truly begins not at 10 cm, but when the mother gets a bearing-down feeling or an unmistakable urge to push. Working with your body is productive and rewarding. Working against your body increases pain and discomfort. Just like learning to swim, you can learn how to give birth. Don't push until you feel a strong need - the clock "starts" when you start pushing.

Each labor is different. Second stage can be very short (only a few minutes), average (around 2 hours), or long (5 hours or more). The vast majority of <u>unmedicated</u> mothers can give birth without mechanical assistance. Giving birth can be an exhilarating experience, sometimes one of joy beyond belief. The actual pushing produces a baby, *your* baby, warm, soft, wet, slippery and real.

GENERAL ASSIGNMENTS

- ☐ Practice relaxation: daily.
- ☐ Complete B.E.S.T. questions: page 97-98.
- ☐ Continue good nutrition and exercises.
- ☐ Birth place tour - page 101-102.
- ☐ Walk 25 min 2X a day.
- ☐ *Husband-Coached Childbirth:* chapters 21-24.
- ☐ Student Center: www.bradleybirth.com

WARMTH RELAXATION

This technique also deals with mental relaxation. You can use it in various positions and with various physical relaxation techniques. Once comfortable and physically relaxed, work on mental relaxation by saying something like this: "Think about the baby, lying in your uterus warm, comfortable, and relaxed. Feel the warmth slowly radiating from your uterus and flowing through your back, down your hips, legs, knees, thighs, ankles, feet, and toes." Stop at each point and talk about the warmth. Talk about sinking deeper and deeper into the bed as she becomes warmer and warmer and more relaxed. Then go back to the uterus again and talk about the warmth moving up her back. Have her feel the warmth spreading to every vertebra, then across her shoulders, arms, hands, and fingers, the back of her neck, her head, face, and jaw. Now her whole body should feel warm and relaxed.

Class 1
Class 2
Class 3
Class 4
Class 5
Class 6
Class 7
Class 8
Class 9
Class 10
Class 11
Class 12

CREATING A POSITIVE ENVIRONMENT IN LABOR

Consider Before Leaving Home

- Don't go in too soon.
- Bring a copy of your pre-admittance papers.
- Bring food.

Upon Arrival At Your Birth Place

- Use first names - they are friendlier.
- Be polite.
- Brief the nurse.
- Answer questions happily and completely.
- Give them a copy of your well-written birth plan.

Getting Started

- Ask for what you need (ice chips, a chair, extra pillows, etc.).
- Set up the environment she needs (music, dim lights, temperature control, privacy, quiet, relaxed).

Tell Them What They Can Do To Help

- "We would appreciate it if you could . . ."
- "It would be helpful if you would . . ."

Offer Sincere Appreciation

- "Thank you for . . ."
- "We appreciate your help!"
- "Thanks!"

Give Them A Reputation To Live Up To

- "I know we're in good hands here."
- "This is a great hospital, that's why we're here!"
- "You're so kind and gentle, you're a great nurse!"

State Your Preferences In A Positive Way

- "We are looking forward to . . ."
- "It is important to us that . . ."
- "Please understand, we feel strongly about . . ."

If Saying No, Say It Nicely

- Use a positive attitude. We're all on the same team.
- "Thank you for your suggestion. We prefer . . ."
- "We feel . . ."

During Contractions In Hard Labor, Protect Her From Being Disturbed

1. Always announce who's there.
2. Say to them:
   "Isn't she doing great!"
   Repeat this many times.
3. Use hand "Stop Sign" and whisper "one moment please."
   If they continue into room, hold up index finger as you say "one moment please" then hand "Stop Sign" and say "I just got her settled".
4. Give her lots of verbal coaching.
5. Complete the contraction with her. (praise, a sip of water, etc.)
6. "Thank you for waiting. How can I help you?"

Stay Calm

- Excitement or fear, can cause extra production of adrenalin. This could cause even natural labor to become ineffective, more painful, or even stop.

Stay Hydrated

- Dehydration can cause a change in blood pressure, temperature and pulse along with a drop in energy output.

Class 1 | Class 2 | Class 3 | Class 4 | Class 5 | Class 6 | Class 7 | Class 8 | Class 9 | **Class 10** | Class 11 | Class 12

LABOR REHEARSAL REVIEW NOTES

Information on this page was introduced throughout classes 1-9
Classes 10, 11, and 12 have labor rehearsals using these techniques

Coach's Check List
(from Class 5)

1. Position
2. Relaxation
3. Rub back
4. Guide breathing
5. Pressure (for practice only)
6. Time contractions
7. Talk her through contraction

Mom's Check List
(from Video: *Bradley on Birthing*)

Sleep Imitation (eyes closed)
1. Do not move during a contraction
2. Abdominal breathing
3. Relaxation
4. "Duh" look (relaxed face)

POSITIONS IN LABOR

Remember the goal of labor is birth. Positions which slow labor down or make labor less effective may prolong the process. Welcome the power of the contractions. Trade off positions: side, bathroom, walking, bathroom, chair, etc. Find what works for you. When standing, bend knees slightly, release back and bottom.

Total Relaxation	Upright	Sitting	Other
Class 1-6 • Side • Contour (requires support under knees & arms) 　• Bed 　• Recliner 　• Bathtub 　• Labor bed	**Class 7-9** Bend knees- release bottom • Lean side against a wall • Lean against coach • Lean back against wall • Lean forward • Labor dance • Walking dance • (Mummy-like) in shower	**Class 7-9** • Chair • Car • Toilet 　• Backward 　• Forward • Front • Against coach • Rocking chair	**Class 7-9** • Pelvic rock 　• over raised labor bed 　• over couch 　• over coach • Asymmetric - one foot up on chair, step stool, step; or on the floor, one knee up, one knee down

COACHING

Verbal Coaching

10 sec - Let it go.

15 sec - Announce seconds:
  Words of relaxation.

30 sec - Announce seconds:
  Words of encouragement.

45 sec - Announce time:
  Words of encouragement.

60 sec - It has been more than 60 seconds.
  Stay still and relaxed until the contraction is over.
  (Never say "the contraction is over")

Talking about Contractions

- Welcome the power of the contraction.
- The stronger the contraction the sooner the birth.
- Let's take one contraction at a time.
- Strong/powerful.
- Effective/efficient.
- Productive.
- Good/positive.
- Opportunity to progress.
- Brings us closer to the birth.
- A gift to our baby.

Tips for Back Labor

Freedom of position is important:
- Side
- Tailor Sit
- Pelvic Rock
- Lean Forward - sitting or standing
- Shower

Pressure:
- Counter pressure on aching area
- Back pressure with: hand, fingertips, fist, palm
- Butt massage
- Light/gentle rub
- Sacrum points

Coach puts pressure on Mom's hand instead of Mom pressing on Coach.
- Hot & Cold compresses
- Hot water bottle
- Corn/rice bag, Face cloth, Ice chips
- Cloth

After the Contraction

Words of praise:
  Great job!

  I'm proud of you!

  You can do it!

  You are doing it!

Help her adjust position: sit up, stand up, etc.
Sip of water, clean-up, reassure.
Walk, rest, dance position, guide, protect, she sets the pace, shower, stretch, etc.
Get ready for next contraction.

Comfort Measures for the Mom

- Cool cloth
- Warm towel
- Hot water bottle
- Massage oil
- Honey
- Lollipop
- Food
- Soup
- Water
- Soft blanket
- Special pillow

Protect Yourself

- Wear comfortable clothes.
- Wear supportive shoes.
- Stand with feet apart and brace yourself.
- Bend your knees when holding her.
- Place yourself with your back against a wall for support.
- Eat.
- Drink water.
- Go to the bathroom.

Class 1
Class 2
Class 3
Class 4
Class 5
Class 6
Class 7
Class 8
Class 9
Class 10
Class 11
Class 12

Class 1
Class 2
Class 3
Class 4
Class 5
Class 6
Class 7
Class 8
Class 9
Class 10
Class 11
Class 12

RELAXATION TECHNIQUES

PHYSICAL RELAXATION

When the uterus contracts it moves forward putting the baby in the proper alignment with the pelvis. If the abdominal muscles are tense this will cause unnecessary pain and discomfort to the mother. Ask someone else to apply pressure to your upper arm while it is relaxed. Then make a fist and bend the arm toward your shoulder. Notice the difference in feeling. The same type of thing happens in labor when tension is present.

Stroking (from/to):	Massage:	Pressure:
• Shoulder • Upper Arm • Elbow • Forearm • Wrist • Hand • Hip • Thigh • Knee • Calf • Ankle • Foot • Top of head • Down hair	• Hands • Feet • Belly • Back • Neck • Shoulders	• Hip squeeze • Palm on coccyx • Fist on sacrum • Tennis balls - place 2 in pantyhose. Use on either side of spine. • Water bottle for back, neck, etc. • Rice or corn bags (heat or freeze). Use against wall, contour position, back or feet. • Thumb pressure on either side of sacrum

MENTAL RELAXATION

What you think about can make a big difference in your level of relaxation. Mental stress can cause physical stress, which can lead to pain and discomfort. Thinking about something pleasant and relaxing is the key. A place you have been, or time you have shared (ocean, mountains, home, holding your new baby, etc.). Imagine what you could see, feel, hear, touch, and smell. Imagine the peace, quiet and safety of this experience.

EMOTIONAL RELAXATION

Perhaps the most important relaxation is emotional relaxation. This means how you feel. It should include a feeling of confidence, safety, and security. Can you depend on your coach? Can you depend on your health care provider? Are you confident about your birthing choices? Have you discussed and do you feel good about your birthing plans? Now let go and relax! You have your basic plan and your back-up for variations.

WORKING WITH YOUR BODY
Study Guide

PREPARATION FOR BIRTH

1. How can the following things help women to prepare to give birth?
   Good nutrition:

   Regular physical exercise:

   Frequent pelvic rocking:

   Doing Kegels regularly:

   Doing lots of squatting:

2. What should the mother and coach practice during pregnancy so that they can be comfortable and confident when it is time to push?

3. What can be done during pregnancy to help decrease the need for an episiotomy and the likelihood of a tear?

4. What can be done ahead of time to help avoid unnecessary pain in second stage?

TRANSITION

1. What are the typical characteristics of transition?
   Possible physical signs:

   Possible emotional signs:

2. How often do women have difficult transitions?

3. What can you do to handle a difficult transition?

THE URGE TO PUSH

1. List four ways that you might recognize the urge to push:

2. How can you differentiate between an overwhelming urge to push, a mild urge to push, and a wishful urge to push?

3. What could you do if the mother has a mild or wishful urge to push but is not completely dilated?

4. What could you do if the mother has an overwhelming urge to push but is not completely dilated?

SECOND STAGE

1. What are the typical characteristics of second stage?

2. What can be done to handle pain in second stage?

3. What positions could the mother assume during second stage?

4. Which position can be used to increase the opening at the outlet of the pelvis by more than 10%?

5. Which position could be the most difficult to give birth in?

6. Which position is most commonly used in the delivery room or birthing bed?

7. No matter which position you choose, there are three things that the mother can do to control pain and increase the effectiveness of each push:

    A. Knees back (elbows up and out) - Why is this important?

    B. Chin on chest - Why is this important?

    C. Curved spine (do not arch your back) - Why is this important?

8. What is the pattern of breath control that is typically used in second stage?

9. During second stage the mother should hold her breath as long as is _____.

10. During second stage the mother should push to the point of _____.

11. What are the coach's responsibilities during second stage?

12. What are the mother's responsibilities during second stage?

13. What sensations may the mother feel during second stage?

14. What are the advantages and disadvantages of episiotomies?
        Advantages: Disadvantages:

Class 1 Class 2 Class 3 Class 4 Class 5 Class 6 Class 7 Class 8 Class 9 Class 10 Class 11 Class 12

15. What can be done during second stage to decrease the need for an episiotomy and to avoid tearing?
- knees back w/ elbows up & out   - be willing to wait a couple more contractions
- push only as body tells you   - push w/ contractions not during rest intervals
                                  - warm compress / perineal massage

16. What is a pressure episiotomy?

17. What conditions should be met before a pressure episiotomy is done?
- baby crowning, mom pushing, skin on perineum is white

18. When done correctly, can the mother feel a pressure episiotomy?

THIRD STAGE

1. If it is necessary to give the mother a local anesthetic to repair an episiotomy or a tear, what may you want to do first so that the drug will not reach the baby?

2. American Academy of Pediatrics, Press Release; July 6, 1999. "If the cord clamping is done too soon after birth, the infant may be deprvied of a placental blood transfusion resulting in lower blood volume and increased risk for anemia later in life... ."

3. What is the physical and emotional importance to the mother and baby of putting the baby to the breast immediately after birth?

4. What is bonding and why is it important?

5. How long may it take for the placenta to be born? 5-45min after birth
- encourage baby to nurse - helps more contractions

6. What may the mother do to help expel the placenta? - nurse

7. List four reasons for the mother to drink orange juice after the baby is born:

8. What criteria should be met before walking soon after the birth?
- mom should not have any nausea   - be breastfeeding   - drinking fluids
- natural birth   - feel good sitting & standing

9. What is the importance of walking soon after the baby is born?
- helps restore circulation   - expels blood clots
realign organs

10. How long will you continue to have contractions after the baby is born? up to 4 weeks after birth happens during breastfeeding

11. What can you do to handle discomfort from after-birth contractions?

12. If you have stitches, what can be applied to your perineum during the first 24 hours to reduce swelling?
- ice / cold packs

13. How can Kegel exercises help the healing of your perineum?
- pull together the tissue aiding in healing

14. When can you start taking sitz baths to ease discomfort and encourage healing?
around 2nd day postpartum

CLASS 11 *(week 11 of 12)*

BEING A GREAT COACH

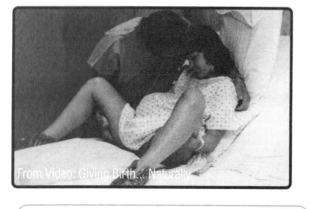

From Video: Giving Birth... Naturally

ABC: alternative birth center.
BOW: bag of waters.
BP: blood pressure.
EFM: electronic fetal monitoring.
LDR: labor, delivery, recovery... a multipurpose hospital room.
LOA: left occiput anterior.
NPO: from the latin "non per os" nothing by mouth; withholding of food and liquid.
OP: occiput posterior, baby's occipital bone (back of head) toward mother's back; "sunny-side-up". Causes "back labor".
PE: pressure episiotomy.
PROM: premature rupture of membranes.
AROM: artificial rupture of membranes.

"The mother has learned how to work with her body in labor and has physically prepared her birthing muscles. You, as the coach, have learned to understand the what, how and why of labor. This will enable you to coach, guide, and encourage her in her ennobling work. You should be well acquainted in advance with her appearance in the various stages of labor. By being prepared for her objective appearance, not only will you feel serene and self-confident through familiarity, but you will be able to apply this knowledge by acting as her coach to actually see to it that things go smoothly. She, in turn, will feel secure in knowing that her ever-present coach not only loves her, but knows what she is about and how to guide her."

From *Husband-Coached Childbirth*

Coaching is very rewarding, but very challenging, physically and emotionally. The mother may be doing the hardest work of her life. Coaches should work on long-term good nutrition, physical activity, relaxation, and mental preparation.

GENERAL ASSIGNMENTS

☐ Kegel: 200 each day.

☐ Continue good nutrition & exercise.

☐ Go through the workbook and complete any unfinished sections.

☐ Practice relaxation 20 min. 2X a day.

☐ Practice together every day.

☐ Walk 30 min + 25 min a day.

☐ Fill out *Student Workbook*, page 89-90.

☐ Read *Student Workbook*, page 93-96.

☐ Coach fill out *Student Workbook*, page 97-98.

☐ Student Center: www.bradleybirth.com

SENSORY RECALL

To practice this weeks technique, begin by either remembering a pleasant experience from your past (i.e. a vacation, a special holiday, something from your childhood, even what it feels like when you crawl in bed after a long, hard day) or actually go to a peaceful, relaxing place. As the mother relaxes, guide her through this experience recalling all of the five senses. Encourage her to remember even the finest details of what she saw. Allow her plenty of time to explore this sense before moving on to the next one. Slowly work through the senses from seeing to touching, hearing, tasting, smelling, and finally have her concentrate on the overall feelings and impressions she associates with this experience. Work this technique every day this week in order to master it. This technique can be very effective during practice and can be useful at any stage in labor.

Class 1
Class 2
Class 3
Class 4
Class 5
Class 6
Class 7
Class 8
Class 9
Class 10
Class 11
Class 12

COACH'S READINESS CHECKLIST

I. CLASSES - Have you attended the full series of Bradley® classes and covered all of the sections in this book including:

Yes No   *How could you improve?*

❑ ❑ Introduction to The Bradley Method®?   _____

❑ ❑ Nutrition?   _____

❑ ❑ Pregnancy?   _____

❑ ❑ Coach's role?   _____

❑ ❑ First stage labor, how your body works?   _____

❑ ❑ Second stage labor, how your body works?   _____

❑ ❑ Planning your labor and birth?   _____

❑ ❑ Variations and unexpected situations?   _____

❑ ❑ Postpartum care?   _____

❑ ❑ First stage labor, how you can work with your body?   _____

❑ ❑ Second stage labor, how you can work with your body? _____

❑ ❑ Coaching?   _____

❑ ❑ Are you ready?   _____

❑ ❑ Your new family?   _____

II. READING - Have you finished reading:

❑ ❑ *Husband-Coached Childbirth?*   _____

❑ ❑ *Children at Birth?*   _____

❑ ❑ *The Womanly Art of Breastfeeding?*   _____

❑ ❑ *Assistant Coach's Manual?*   _____

❑ ❑ *Natural Childbirth the Bradley® Way?*   _____

❑ ❑ Quick Reference Guide for Coaches?   _____

❑ ❑ Coaching Cues?   _____

❑ ❑ B.E.S.T (Bradley® Energy-Saving Techniques) article?   _____

III. ASSIGNMENTS - Have you completed your:

❑ ❑ Birth plan?   _____

❑ ❑ First stage study guide?   _____

Class 1 | Class 2 | Class 3 | Class 4 | Class 5 | Class 6 | Class 7 | Class 8 | Class 9 | Class 10 | **Class 11** | Class 12

❑ ❑ Second stage study guide? _____

❑ ❑ Cesarean choices? _____

❑ ❑ Birth place visit? _____

❑ ❑ B.E.S.T. fill-in page? _____

❑ ❑ Reference information? _____

IV. PRACTICE AND PREPARATION FOR LABOR - Have you:

❑ ❑ Practiced relaxation techniques every day for at least 20 minutes? _____

❑ ❑ Mastered all of the relaxation techniques taught in class? _____

❑ ❑ Become comfortable relaxing in various positions and situations? _____

❑ ❑ Encouraged her to do everything she can to stay healthy and low risk? _____

❑ ❑ Built a good rapport with your birth team? _____

❑ ❑ Planned activities to pass the time in early labor? _____

❑ ❑ Arranged for time off work to be with your partner during labor, no matter when it begins or how long it takes? _____

❑ ❑ Been careful to get plenty of rest in case labor begins soon? _____

❑ ❑ Done what you can to avoid excess stress? _____

❑ ❑ Been a positive reassuring influence on your partner? _____

V. COACH'S PREPARATION FOR POSTPARTUM - Have you:

❑ ❑ Arranged for a paternity leave (1-2 weeks to be together as a family)? _____

❑ ❑ Prepared to take care of all household responsibilities for at least two weeks (or arranged for someone else to do it)? _____

❑ ❑ Considered ways you can be involved with taking care of the baby? _____

❑ ❑ Considered what you might say if anyone criticizes the way that you have chosen to parent your baby? _____

❑ ❑ Prepared a list of things that people could do to help if they offer? _____

❑ ❑ Considered how your relationship with your wife will change and how you can help this to be positive? _____

❑ ❑ Written a letter to your new baby detailing how you feel now and what you are doing to prepare for his/her birth? _____

Class 1
Class 2
Class 3
Class 4
Class 5
Class 6
Class 7
Class 8
Class 9
Class 10
Class 11
Class 12

WHOSE JOB IS IT?

For each job, please write in whose responsibility it is. Indicate whether it is something the mother, coach, nurse, midwife, doctor, or family needs to do.

1. Who will go with the mother to classes to learn what to expect and how to help her in labor? — coach

2. Who will encourage her to exercise during pregnancy?

3. Who will encourage her to eat well every day?

4. Who will help her to avoid and alleviate stress?

5. Who will help her practice relaxation every day?

6. Who will help her during pre-labor contractions?

7. Who will help her in early labor?

8. Who will fix her some food in early labor?

9. Who will encourage her to keep drinking?

10. Who will call the doctor or midwife when she's in labor? — coach

11. Who will carry the bags to the car?

12. Who will help get her to the car?

13. Who will drive her to the birth place?

14. Who will sign the admitting forms and answer questions?

15. Who will set up a peaceful environment?

16. Who will keep her relaxed?

17. Who will remind her to slow her breathing and relax again after something disturbs her?

18. Who will encourage her?

19. Who will recognize the natural alignment plateau and keep her from getting discouraged?

20. Who will spoon ice chips into her mouth? — coach

21. Who will wipe her sweaty brow?

22. Who will dim the lights?

23. Who will keep people from interrupting her?

24. Who will convince her to go to the bathroom often even if she is afraid to get out of bed?

25. Who will she rely on to keep watch and help her to avoid unnecessary pain?

26. Who will she depend on to tell her she's doing a great job over and over and over and over again?

27. Who will convince her to get up and walk around if she needs to?

28. Who will walk her up and down the halls, back and forth, for hours, if necessary?

29. Who will remind her why she's doing this so that she can go on, even if she's in a lot of pain?

30. Who will act as an advocate for the mother when decisions must be made?

31. Who will know what relaxes her?

32. Who will know when it's time to try a different relaxation technique?

33. Who will know which techniques work best for her?

34. Who will praise her?

35. Who will massage her feet?

36. Who will rub her sore back?

37. Who will hold her up in the shower if she wants to take one?

38. Who will tell the birth team when she needs to push?

39. Who will help her find a good pushing position?

40. Who will hold her up in the pushing position, even for hours, if necessary?

41. Who will remind her to push to the point of comfort?

42. Who will remind her to hold her breath only as long as is comfortable?

43. Who will make sure that the baby's head is crowning and the mother is pushing, if a pressure episiotomy is done?

44. Who will tell her he can see the head?

45. Who will share those last few important minutes before the baby is born?

46. Who will help the birth attendant by bringing the baby up to the mother's breast?

47. Who will share the special time of bonding?

48. Who will cut the cord?

49. Who will tell the family that the baby has arrived?

50. Who will the mother say she couldn't have done it without?

Note: Teacher, have bold questions read in class.

Class 1
Class 2
Class 3
Class 4
Class 5
Class 6
Class 7
Class 8
Class 9
Class 10
Class 11
Class 12

ARE YOU READY?

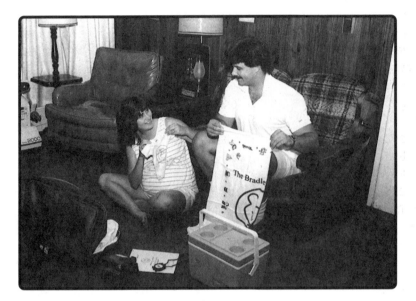

Are you ready? Having a baby is an athletic event, much like swimming. If someone were to say that in nine months he was going to throw you into ten feet of water, you would want to learn how to swim. Being pregnant, the same rules apply. If you know that at the end of nine months you are going to give birth, you should learn how. If you don't, you will be like a rock that sinks when thrown in the water. If you do, you will be like the fish that floats and swims with ease.

B.E.S.T.: Bradley® energy-saving techniques.

Emotional signpost: emotional state which helps predict the stage of labor a mother is in.

Hawthorne effect: the effect of personal attention, seen in industrial engineering, as well as in labor.

Duration: how long contractions last.

Emergency childbirth: birth in other than the expected place, or with other than the expected people. May well be normal, natural and safe... don't panic.

Frequency: how often contractions occur. Time from the beginning of one to the beginning of the next one.

Intensity: how strong contractions are.

Intrauterine life: the entire period of pregnancy from the time the fertilized baby enters the uterus until birth.

Malar flush: a reddish color of the cheeks, typical of the onset of labor... but not always.

Modesty: not displaying one's body... a condition which gradually disappears during labor... one sign of progress is less concern for one's clothing.

The B.E.S.T. Way to Handle Your Labor!

The following is a list of energy-saving techniques which thousands of women have found effective and useful during labor. No one knows how long she will be in labor; so, it is always best to plan on doing everything you can to conserve energy from the very beginning. Even if you end up having a fairly short labor, you will find that you still use up a tremendous amount of energy. Many obstetricians endorse these suggestions but each labor is unique, check with your own birth team. Remember, medical interventions (including cesareans) often become necessary during the course of labors due to exhaustion caused by wasted energy.

A. Don't pay attention too soon.

Most women experience many series of contractions throughout the weeks and months prior to their actual labors. These natural pregnancy contractions are an important and beneficial part of your body's preparation for birth. It is often a challenge late in pregnancy to determine whether the contractions you are experiencing are natural pregnancy contractions (NPC), which mean your body is preparing for labor, or natural labor contractions (NLC), which mean you are in labor.

It is important that you don't waste your precious energy getting all excited and perhaps even losing sleep over the natural pregnancy contractions. These NPC's are a very important part of your body's preparing itself for labor, but are nothing to become alarmed about. Generally, you should not concern yourself with contractions until they are: 10 minutes apart or less, lasting approximately 60 seconds, and are strong enough that you don't move or talk during contractions. These natural labor contractions should gradually become stronger and closer together, and often continue, regardless of change in activity. To get an idea of how strong your contractions are, you can ask yourself, "If I were in the middle of the street and a contraction started, would I have to stop for the contraction?" They will become this strong during the natural course of most labors.

When your situation meets all these criteria, then you are probably, but not definitely, in labor. If you are planning a birth center or hospital birth, it is probably not time to go there yet. It is generally better to wait until the labor is well-established and mother is in hard labor before leaving. These are general guide-lines which apply to most labors although each situation varies. You should check with your birth team for their suggestions too.

B. Face your labor calmly.

When you think you might be in labor, eat something, have something to drink, go for a walk, take a warm shower, and then take a nap. If these are natural pregnancy contractions, they will probably subside by the time you've done all this. If your contractions continue, stay calm and follow your normal daily routine as long as possible. Remember, adrenalin which comes from excitement, can cause even natural labor contractions to become ineffective, more painful, or even stop.

C. Go back home if you arrive at your birth place too early.

Most first-time parents end up going to their birth place once or twice before their real labor starts. As Dr. Bradley explains, "It's not that you are crazy or that you're not quite bright; your medical team probably won't know if you're in labor, either. They will observe you for a while to see if your labor continues and if you progress." Try not to be too over-anxious or concerned. If you're not sure whether or not you're in labor, call your Bradley® teacher or your birth team and discuss it. The only way to know for sure if these are natural pregnancy contractions or natural labor contractions is to wait and see if the baby is born. Then you'll know for sure that it was labor.

Regardless of which type of contractions you're having, you need coaching and you need support. You may wish to meet your birth attendant at the office instead of at the hospital, if you are concerned about arriving too early. If you do go to the hospital to be checked, you might consider getting checked only; that is, wait to be admitted, to have blood and urine tests, to put on a hospital gown, etc. Once you've gone through all those procedures, you are emotionally committed and will want to stay, even if the hospital staff is encouraging you to go home.

Dr. Victor Berman a well-known obstetrician who specializes in natural childbirth, encourages women to follow what is known as "Berman's Law," which says that most women should not stay in the hospital if they are less than five centimeters dilated. This is a very good guideline, most of the time. If you are less than five centimeters and still showing early labor signs (both physical and behavioral), then you are probably too early, especially since most hospitals impose time limits for labor and birth. Once in a rare while, a woman is three or four centimeters, going on second stage. In this case, you would know from her physical and behavioral signs that it doesn't matter what her cervix is saying - she's about to have a baby. Under these circumstances, you might choose to stay a while.

D. Use relaxation to handle contractions.

Tensing up during contractions will waste valuable energy and can cause a tremendous amount of totally unnecessary pain. It is much better to use deep relaxation techniques, which are more effective and less painful. Relaxation should have been practiced during pregnancy. Women should strive to be so good at relaxing that they can automatically relax completely as contractions begin and in response to their coach's voice and touch.

Relaxation is the key to labor and can be very helpful even for women who have not practiced much, prior to labor. But, it is the couple who has faithfully practiced and really mastered the relaxation techniques taught in class who can realize fully the incredible benefits of deep relaxation in labor.

E. Use normal abdominal breathing during labor.

You know how to breathe already. You have been doing a good job of it all of your life. Your breathing automatically becomes more rapid when you've been exerting a lot of energy. It automatically slows when you are calm and relaxed. You have not had to worry about adjusting your breathing through the many situations you've faced in your life and there is no reason to start now. Your breathing will automatically adjust itself in labor too.

Chest-breathing and altered breathing patterns use up a tremendous amount of energy, and are more likely to cause hyperventilation, which has been shown to be dangerous for both the mother and baby. "Breathing" is not as effective as relaxation to deal with contractions. So, relax and let your breathing take care of itself.

F. Walk during labor.

Dr. Roberto Caldeyro-Barcia has studied walking during labor and found that it shortens labor by an average of 28%. Walking opens the inlet of the pelvis, so the baby has more room to get down into and maneuver through the pelvis. Women also seem to have more energy and experience less pain when they are up and around than when they've been lying down for a long time. Get up and walk around-you'll be glad you did!

G. Keep drinking during labor.

Most birth teams we've worked with encourage women to keep drinking in labor because drinking a large glass of water or juice every hour helps to replace fluids, prevent dehydration and keep the body functioning properly. While in labor, each woman is doing, perhaps, the hardest work of her life. Giving birth is an athletic event. The body depends on fluids to keep it functioning properly. A lot of fluids are lost through perspiration and discharge. It is important to avoid becoming dehydrated.

Dehydration during labor can cause a woman's blood pressure to change, her temperature to rise, her pulse rate to increase-all clearly undesirable conditions in labor.

H. Eat if you're hungry.

Eating is a very important way to restore energy and to keep up your strength. You will be using up a tremendous amount of energy in labor. Tune-in to your body. Ask yourself, "Am I hungry?" and, "What am I hungry for?" Eating will often cause natural pregnancy contractions to subside and is thought to prevent premature labor.

Many women are quite hungry in early labor. They eat a good meal and have the strength to labor for hours, then go on to give birth to their babies. Once in hard labor, most women are no longer hungry in which case they probably should not eat.

Some hospitals still restrict food intake of mothers in labor. If a mother needs some extra energy in hard labor some juice, hard candy, or a spoonful of honey may do the trick.

I. Sleep if you're sleepy.

No one knows how long she will be in labor. If you can sleep then sleep. You will need the energy! Sleep between contractions.

If you are having regular contractions, have your coach wake you a few seconds or so before the next contraction starts so that you have some warning that the contraction is coming and you won't wake up at the peak.

Do not be afraid to sleep during labor. Good strong contractions will wake you, and we don't know of any unmedicated mother who ever slept through having a baby. Some labors may progress slowly because the mother is tired and needs some sleep.

We know many mothers who went through long first stages; but, during transition, their contractions stopped completely. These mothers took this opportunity to get some rest. Most of them slept for about two hours. When they awoke, they felt refreshed and went immediately into second stage and pushed their babies out.

If you find that you're very tired in second stage you can sleep between contractions, then, too. You'll be glad you did!

J. Stay active as long as you can.

Just because you are in labor is no reason to lie down and act sick. Just because you have been assigned a hospital bed is no reason to feel you have to be there all the time.

The side relaxation position should only be used if the contractions have become so strong that you must lie down and concentrate on relaxation or if you are tired and need to sleep.

Keep yourself occupied with games, books, music, or whatever you enjoy doing. Going for a walk outside and taking a bath or shower are often invigorating for women in labor. Lying down for long periods of time can cause a mother to become bored and tired, and that's not a good thing in labor.

Sure, labor is a lot of very hard work; but it can be fun, too! Enjoy this precious time as you labor to give birth to your baby.

K. Try taking a warm bath or shower.

When you're really getting down to hard labor, perhaps just before you leave for your birth place, you might want to try getting in warm water, provided the bag of waters is still intact and the temperature does not exceed body temperature. This often reduces pain, encourages deep relaxation, and speeds labor. Being submerged in warm water seems to help women "let go" an important part of giving birth. So for labor, when the going gets tough, the tough take a bath!

L. Avoid taking medication.

The drugs and medications used in childbirth today are neither as safe nor as effective as most people believe. They pose a definite danger to the mother and the baby, and are not necessary for the vast majority of couples who take Bradley® classes.

Taking medication during labor can be a waste of time and energy. The most common drug used in childbirth today is Demerol®. Although often refered to as "just a little relaxer," it is not as harmless as it sounds. Demerol® is a narcotic, the same family as heroin. Besides its many effects on the mother and baby, Demerol® relaxes the uterus. Think about that for a minute. Is this what you want to do in labor? Your uterus is a large bag of muscles which contract to open the cervix and expel the baby. Relaxing the uterus is likely to slow the progress of labor. Often, the medication leaves a mother groggy and unable to handle her contractions well; therefore, she experiences more pain. Sometimes mothers who take medication must wait until it wears off before they can continue progressing.

Taking medication in labor is quite a risk and is best left for the case of a complication where the benefits outweigh the risks.

Dr. Bradley says, "The loving encouragement from a trained coach can do more for the comfort and relaxation of his wife than any amount of medication." So keep up the good coaching, and avoid the medication.

M. Continued enthusiastic encouragement is essential.

Allowing yourselves to become depressed or discouraged is the worst thing you can do! The work you are doing is extremely important. Yes, it's difficult and, perhaps, quite painful, but it is important! Your baby needs this labor and you are the only one who can give it to him. You need this labor too; don't sell yourself short! You can do it! You are doing it! Just hang on!

Get the most out of every contraction by completely relaxing and letting go. Don't become discouraged because of slow or stalled dilation. Remember the natural alignment plateau. There is much more to your labor than mere dilation.

Don't get hung up on time. Instead of saying to yourself, "I've been in labor for two days now." say, "I've been in hard labor for three hours." Okay, maybe you have been in labor for two days. However, if you've been careful to follow these guidelines and conserve your energy, you've had two days with lots of rest and plenty of support and attention from your coach (and contractions once-in-a- while). You're ready and able to face the hard work in front of you. How long have you been in active labor with strong, all-encompassing contractions and definite active labor behavioral signs? That's all you need to think about.

Are you fine, physically? Are the baby's vital signs good? As long as there are no clear indications of a complication and you are careful to conserve your energy, you can continue to follow the natural course of your labor.

Allowing your labor to follow its natural course may not be easy, but don't fool yourself-it does make a difference! You are doing the best thing for you and your baby. The two of you would not be as well off with some medication or a cesarean section done for no reason. This is the only chance you will have to give birth to this baby. You will not be in labor forever. Soon you will be able to rest. Allowing your labor to follow it's natural course is so important.

There are good reasons for everything in nature and there are good reasons for your long labor. Every minute is worthwhile. Every contraction is beneficial. You are doing, perhaps, the most important work a human being can do in her life and you deserve all the credit and praise in the world.

N. Be aware of natural, effective techniques to speed labor.

Sometimes labors go on and on, which is probably beneficial as long as people are patient and the mother is careful to conserve her energy. If it becomes necessary to speed the labor for some reason, there are a few very effective techniques you can use: 1) Get up and walk. Walking opens the inlet of the pelvis to get the baby down and is an effective means of speeding labor. 2) Use nipple stimulation. Just use your fingers or the heel of your hand and rub up and down over your nipple. Right through your gown is fine. Nipple stimulation has been shown to be an effective way to accelerate labor, and has been used for centuries. Nipple stimulation usually results in more powerful, more frequent contractions almost immediately. Continue using stimulation between each contraction, as long as is necessary. 3) Another means of accelerating labor is to use acupressure. Push your thumb up against the palate (the roof of your mouth), an action similar to sucking your thumb. 4) Do what is necessary to reduce the mother's fears and anxieties. Sometimes, all that she needs is to discuss her fears and be assured that she is not alone. Some mothers who go to the hospital too soon and find that they can't relax well there may need to go home for a while so that they can "give in" and let labor take over. Other mothers find that they are so uneasy at home that they cannot relax well and "give in" to their labors until they are in the hospital. Each situation must be evaluated individually.

So, if it becomes necessary to speed labor, first talk with the mother. Find out if any changes are necessary so that she can: fully relax, "give in" to her labor, let her body open up and give birth to her baby. Then, recharge the mother in some way (a spoonful of honey, a cool drink, a warm shower, for example). Instill in her a positive, enthusiastic attitude. It is time to get down to work and have this baby! Next, go for a walk outside, around the corridors... someplace as spacious and private as possible. Most mothers do not like feeling confined, and feel strange rubbing their nipples and sucking their thumb in public.

As you walk do some nipple stimulation, suck your thumb briefly; then you will most likely have a contraction. Lean forward against your coach. Let your coach support you. You just hang loose and limp, completely relaxed, and concentrate on letting go and opening up. Each contraction should be followed by enthusiastic encouragement. (We're really getting somewhere! You are doing a great job! You look great! Let's do it again!)

Then do some more walking at a good pace, nipple stimulation, and thumb sucking, resulting in another good, strong, effective contraction. The mother will probably be having contractions which are much more powerful now. She may comment that these contractions are more painful, and that's great! The stronger the contractions, the sooner your baby will be born.

These very effective techniques are likely to bring results. Although you may need to continue this way for many hours, changes may also come about very quickly. Watch for the pain which moves lower and lower down her back or down in front against her pubic bone and the feeling of tremendous pressure low in her pelvis. These are all great! They are signs that the baby is coming down. Keep this up with an enthusiastic attitude and continue with these effective techniques. Remind the mother to drink and go to the bathroom often.

Take one contraction at a time and watch for progress.

O. Push only when you're ready to push.

Try not to push until you feel an undeniable urge to push. Many women waste energy pushing before they are ready. Often a mother is encouraged to push too soon (before her urge to push) and the baby is pushed down in a bad position, making a normal delivery difficult or even impossible. When a woman is in hard labor, relaxing and handling her contractions well, perhaps she and her baby need some more time before pushing, even if she is completely dilated.

Once in a while a woman does not recognize her urge to push. She grunts and groans, tenses up, can no longer relax well and has a lot of very painful contractions. In this case. The coach might need to encourage her to try pushing gently and see how it feels.

When done correctly, pushing can be an effective means of pain control. When a mother begins actively pushing, she should be sure that it feels better to push than not to push. On occasion, a woman will give birth without pushing at all. These are all normal variations.

P. Use positive pushing techniques.

1) Push to the point of comfort. Exert only the amount of energy necessary at the time. This is not a contest. Push at your own speed. There are a lot of very important and beneficial processes going on inside of your body right now. It is all right if you take your time. 2) Hold your breath only as long as is comfortable. You may need to take several breaths during a contraction. Your body will let you know how often to breathe. Pay attention and you'll do just fine. 3) While you're pushing, relax everything except the muscles necessary to push and hold yourself in the pushing position you've chosen. Do not: tense your face, clench your jaw, tense your hands or feet, or tense across your buttocks.

"Let go" with each push. Push down and out. Let your body open up. Let your baby come down and out. The perineum should bulge during pushes. 4) Between contractions, let go of your legs, drop your arms, lean back and completely relax. You are likely to have longer rest periods between contractions now. Take advantage of this time and recoup your energy. Some women even doze between contractions and that's fine.

Q. Be aware of effective pushing positions.

Mothers should be free to use whatever pushing position they prefer. If the mother is running out of energy or a time limit is imposed on her, she might need to use one of the most effective pushing positions to speed her second stage.

Squatting opens the outlet of the pelvis by 10- 15%. A modified squat on a delivery table is not quite as effective, but still may be useful. Using a full squat position coupled with breath-holding and positive pushing techniques, is probably the fastest way to push a baby out.

We believe that it is best to allow each labor to follow its natural course, if at all possible. Once in a while these aggressive pushing techniques become important; so all couples should be aware of them.

Have a happy birth-day!

In this article, we have covered each point briefly. To learn more about why The Bradley Method® is unique and how you too can learn to give birth naturally, contact your local Bradley® instructor and have a very happy birth-day!

ARE YOU READY TO DO YOUR B.E.S.T.?

This questionnaire should be filled out by the coach prior to the Coach Card being issued.

B.E.S.T. stands for:

_____ _____ - _____ _____

A. DON'T PAY ATTENTION TOO SOON.

1. What signs will help you to decide whether you are in labor or just having Braxton-Hicks contractions? *-10 min apart or less - regular contractions getting closer together regardless of activity*

2. At what point should you begin timing contractions, in most cases? *-10min apart or less*

3. What signs will you be looking for to help you decide when to leave for your birth place?
Contractions: *continuing even if eat, drink, shower, nap*

Behavioral signs: *more accepting & serious*

Physical signs: *no longer hungry or talkative sweating,*

B. FACE YOUR LABOR CALMLY.

1. When you think you might be in labor, what five things should you do? *1 eat 2 nap 3 walk 4 shower 5 breathe*

2. What can adrenalin/epinephrine (which can come from excitement, fear, anxiety, etc.) do to your labor? *slow it, more painful stop it*

C. GO BACK HOME IF YOU ARRIVE AT YOUR BIRTH PLACE TOO EARLY.

1. Whom should you call to discuss your situation when you think you might be in labor? *Dr.*

2. What does "Berman's Law" say? *physical & behavioral signs show early labor don't stay in hospital if less than 5cm dilated*

D. USE RELAXATION TO HANDLE CONTRAC-TIONS.

1. Tensing up during contractions will waste *energy* and cause *unnecessary* pain.

2. What is the key to The Bradley Method®? *relaxation*

3. Women should *relax* every day and become so good at relaxing that they can

relax completely in response to their coach's *voice* and *touch* .

E. USE NORMAL, ABDOMINAL BREATHING.

1. What are three reasons The Bradley Method® doesn't teach altered breathing patterns? *1 waste energy 2 cause hyperventilation 3 cause tension not relaxed*

2. If you relax and tune-in to your body, your breathing will take care of itself. ☑True.

F. WALK DURING LABOR.

1. Dr. Roberto Caldeyro-Barcia has determined that walking during labor *speeds* labor on an average of 28%.

2. Walking helps to open the pelvis to help the baby come down.

G. KEEP DRINKING DURING LABOR.

1. What does drinking one large glass of liquid every hour during labor help to do? *keep you hydrated, replaces fluids, keeps body functioning, prevents dehydration*

2. List 4 signs of dehydration. *1) high bp 2) rise in temp 3) rise in pulse 4) decreased energy output*

H. EAT IF YOU'RE HUNGRY.

1. Eating during early labor can help you to store *energy* and keep your *strength* up.

2. What two questions can you ask yourself when trying to decide if you should eat? *1) Am I hungry? 2) what am I hungry for? 3) how long since I last ate?*

3. If your intake has been restricted and you feel a need to raise your blood sugar, what can you try? *-clear fluids - 7up, jello, popsicles, honey*

I. SLEEP IF YOU'RE SLEEPY.

1. If you can sleep then *sleep* !

2. What can a coach do for a woman who's sleeping between contractions so that the next contraction does not take her by surprise? *for more active labor rub arm, wake up before it starts,*

3. Do women ever take a break and sleep for an hour or two during the course of a normal labor? *sometimes*

4. Do women ever sleep between contractions in second stage? *sometimes*

©2010 AAHCC

Class 1 Class 2 Class 3 Class 4 Class 5 Class 6 Class 7 Class 8 Class 9 Class 10 **Class 11** Class 12

Last Resort Kit?

J. STAY ACTIVE AS LONG AS YOU CAN.

1. Should a woman in early labor lie down and try not to move? What effect could this have on her labor? *-during the day moving helps labor progress*

2. When should you begin using the side relaxation position? *-when you are tired*

3. What could you do during labor to pass the time and stay active?
- walking   -tv
- showering   -movies
- games   -music

K. TRY TAKING A WARM BATH OR SHOWER.

1. When would it be especially helpful to labor in warm water? *-hard labor*
-before leave for hospital

2. In what case should you check with your birth attendant before taking a bath or going into a spa or hot tub? *-if bag of waters is broken* *ask Dr.*

3. When in a spa or hot tub, it is best to keep the temperature below *body temp*.

4. What does getting into warm water generally do for a woman in labor? *relax's muscles reduces pain can help speed labor*

L. AVOID TAKING MEDICATION.

1. Are there any potentially dangerous side effects to the mother and baby from the drugs which can be used during childbirth? *yes*

2. Do the vast majority of mothers trained in The Bradley Method® need to take medication during labor and/or birth? *90% do not require pain meds*

3. Medication, as well as the various life-saving techniques which can be used in labor, are best left for the case of a true complication where the *benefits* outweigh the *risks*.

4. According to Dr. Bradley, the loving encouragement from a trained coach can do more for the *comfort* and *relaxation* of his wife than any amount of *medication*.

M. CONTINUED ENTHUSIASTIC ENCOURAGEMENT IS ESSENTIAL.

1. What can you do to prevent yourselves from becoming depressed and discouraged during a long labor? *-visualization -rest -rocking chair -blankie*

2. How can you get the most out of every contraction? *-relax and let go -surrender to it*

3. As long as there are no indications of a complication and you are careful to *conserve* your *energy*, you can continue to follow the natural course of your labor.

N. BE AWARE OF NATURAL, EFFECTIVE TECHNIQUES TO SPEED LABOR.

1. List four things that are likely to help speed up labor. *1) walking 3) thumb sucking -chiropractor 2) nipple stim 4) relaxation -make out*

2. What discomforts for the mother are also signs that the baby is coming down? *-pressure in pelvis & lower back*

O. PUSH ONLY WHEN YOU'RE READY TO PUSH

1. Why is it important for the mother to wait for her urge to push? *-avoid tearing -not waste energy -pushing too soon can push baby into a bad position*

2. What guideline can help you to determine if it's time to push? *-feels better pushing than not -has the urge -feels like need to have a bowel mvmt*

P. USE POSITIVE PUSHING TECHNIQUES.

1. During second stage, the mother should push to the point of *comfort* and hold her breath only as long as is *comfortable*.

2. What should the mother do between contractions during second stage? *-relax -let go of legs*

Q. BE AWARE OF THE MOST EFFECTIVE PUSHING POSITIONS.

1. What position can the mother use to open the outlet of the pelvis by more than 10%? *squatting*

2. What other position can also help to open the outlet of the pelvis but is generally more acceptable in a hospital environment? *classic or modified squat*

HAVE A VERY HAPPY BIRTH-DAY!

Note: These suggestions are for normal labors. Thousands of women have used these techniques and found them effective and useful during labor. Many obstetricians endorse these suggestions, but each labor is unique. Check with your own birth team.

Class 1 Class 2 Class 3 Class 4 Class 5 Class 6 Class 7 Class 8 Class 9 Class 10 **Class 11** Class 12

EMERGENCY CHILDBIRTH

The following suggestions were edited from *Emergency Childbirth*, a joint publication of the U.S. Department of Defense, Office of Civil Defense, the U.S. Department of Health, Education and Welfare and the American Medical Association. Although it was first written for families who might have to take refuge in fallout shelters, the same advice could be applied to most emergency births: in the car on the way to the hospital, snowstorms, earthquakes, floods, or any situation which would leave you on your own without medical assistance.

WHAT TO DO

1. Let nature be your best helper. Childbirth is a very natural act.
2. At first signs of labor, assign the best-qualified person to remain with mother. *(Editor's note: a trained husband may be the best qualified.)*
3. Be calm; reassure mother.
4. Place mother and attendant in the most protected place.
5. Have hands as clean as possible.
6. Keep hands away from birth canal.
7. See that baby breathes well.
8. Place baby face down across mother's abdomen.
9. Keep baby warm. *(Editor's note: Dr. Bradley says immediate breastfeeding will help expel the placenta, lower the risk of excessive bleeding, provide warmth [if baby is skin-to-skin with mother] and provide essential immunities for the baby.)*
10. Wrap afterbirth/placenta with baby.
11. Keep baby with mother constantly.
12. Make mother as comfortable as possible.
13. Identify baby.

WHAT NOT TO DO

1. DO NOT hurry.
2. DO NOT pull on the baby; let the baby be born naturally.
3. DO NOT pull on the cord; let the placenta (afterbirth) come naturally.
4. DO NOT tie and cut the cord until baby AND the placenta come naturally.
5. DO NOT give medication.

DO NOT HURRY - LET NATURE TAKE HER COURSE

Every expectant mother and the members of her family should do all they can to prepare for emergency births. They will need to know what to do and what to have ready. The Bradley Method® advocates childbirth education. It does NOT encourage unattended births.

* * *

In additon to the above information, you may wish to read *Emergency Childbirth* by Gregory J. White, M.D.

Each family approaching the time of their child's birth should learn of the emergency medical facilities near their home. Are paramedics available? How do you get them? Which hospitals offer emergency care for mother AND baby? (Watch out - not all hopsitals with an "Emergency Room" sign can deal with obstetrics.)

Class 1 Class 2 Class 3 Class 4 Class 5 Class 6 Class 7 Class 8 Class 9 Class 10 Class 11 Class 12

WHAT IS LABOR?

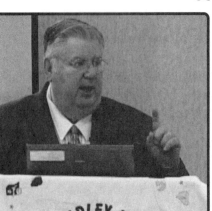

Jay Hathaway, AAHCC, is Co-Executive Director of the American Academy of Husband-Coached Childbirth®. With his wife, Marjie, he has taught over 3,600 couples to give birth. He has trained over 4,000 teachers in The Bradley Method® and has produced over forty films and videos on childbirth and related topics. Jay suggests that many of the problems in obstetrics today are because people do not know and understand what labor is.

What is labor? What is it for? Why have labor, why not just have birth? Contrary to what most people believe, Jay believes that there are some very good reasons for labor and they have little, if anything, to do with cervical dilation.

The following is a list of possible reasons for labor, beginning with the least important first. Write in other important points as you discuss these ideas. This discussion may give you a different perspective on what you are trying to accomplish and why it is important.

I. A warning or signal that a new human life is about to enter the family, community, and this world.

II. A time of physical preparation within and for the mother's body.
    A. To prepare to give birth.

    B. To prepare to become a mother.

III. A physical preparation for the baby's body for being born, changing from an intrauterine life to an extra-uterine life.

IV. A period of time to assist the mother to grow and change psychologically (emotionally and mentally), for giving up the status of "pregnant woman" and for accepting the responsibilities of mothering a newborn.

V. A period of time to assist the baby to grow and change psychologically (emotionally and mentally) for the "first day of the rest of his or her life."

I don't know which, if any, of these points you agree with. I hope that, for at least a few of them, you said to yourself, "Yes, I think that's right." I want to suggest to you that when you are in labor, each of you appreciate that something very important is being done. Nobody else can labor for you. Nobody can give your baby what he/she needs. There are other ways, there are easier ways, but there is no better way than to labor and give birth to your baby naturally.

If you think you're doing something trivial and perhaps not even doing it very well, then labor is much more difficult. If, in the back of your mind, you think you are doing this because your baby needs it, then your labor will become a joy - not easy, not necessarily painless, but extremely worthwhile and rewarding. You can't go back and give birth to this baby over again, so be prepared, dedicated, and keep your baby's needs in mind as you labor.

If you could hold this baby in your arms today for one hour, get to know him, and then put him back inside, there is nothing you wouldn't do for that baby - no job too hard, no pain too intense. If you knew it was for the good of your baby... you could do anything.

BIRTH PLACE TOUR

This form is designed to help you make the move from your home to your birth place as smooth and comfortable as possible. The information is important, whether you use it to become familiar with your planned birth place or your backup birth place.

Use this visit to become familiar and to set up positive communications with the special people you have chosen to be a part of your birth experience. It is not designed to help you choose a birth place; it is to help you become comfortable with the birth place and birth team you have already chosen.

Introduce yourselves (first names are most friendly) and meet as many of the nurses as possible. Record their names in the space provided. Tell them why you have chosen to go there. Be sure they know that you appreciate the attitudes and policies they have which make this a special place to give birth. Be friendly, positive and enthusiastic. When you convey a positive attitude, you become special to the staff and will find them more friendly and supportive in labor. Be sure to pre-register to save time.

Name of birth place:
_____

Address:
_____
_____

Phone number(s):
(   )_____ or (   )_____

Directions:
_____
_____
_____

Alternate route:
_____
_____
_____

Where is the best place to park?
   During the day: _____

   At night: _____

Which entrance should you use?
   During the day: _____

   At night: _____

What admitting procedures can you take care of in advance?
_____
_____
_____

Would they like you to attend any special classes other than your comprehensive Bradley Method® course?
_____

What will need to be taken care of when you arrive in labor? Admitting procedures?
_____
_____

Prepping procedures?
_____
_____

What room will you be in during labor?
_____

Where will you put your belongings?
_____

Where is the bathroom the mother should use?
_____

Where is a bathroom the coach can use?
_____

Can you wear your own clothes during labor?
   Mother_____ Coach_____

Where will you walk during labor?
_____

How will you handle incoming and outgoing calls?
_____
_____

Where can you get something to eat and drink?
_____
_____

Class 1
Class 2
Class 3
Class 4
Class 5
Class 6
Class 7
Class 8
Class 9
Class 10
Class 11
Class 12

Where is the shower or hot tub the mother can use in labor?

_____

Will you need to change rooms when it is time to give birth? If so, where will you move?

_____

At what point would you move?

_____

Will you have to move your belongings? If so, where?

_____

Will the coach have to change his clothes, wear a mask, etc.? If so, where will he get these items and where should he change?

_____

_____

How long will you stay in the same room after the baby is born? _____

When will the family have a chance to bond, undisturbed?

_____

After the birth, will the baby be separated from the parents at any time? If so, why, and where would he/she go?

_____

_____

Will the family be moved into another room after the birth?

_____

If so, where will you be moved?

_____

Where will you put your belongings?

_____

Who will move them?

_____

In the new room, where is the bathroom she should use?

_____

Where can the mother take a shower?

_____

What are the visiting policies?

_____

_____

If you have planned to use a special labor room and it is occupied or your situation changes, where will you be during your labor and birth?

_____

What policies and procedures will be different during labor, in this case?

_____

What will be different during the birth?

_____

_____

What will be different after the baby is born?

_____

_____

How long will you stay after the birth?

_____

What criteria would they like you to meet before going home?

_____

Mother_____

_____

Baby_____

_____

What procedures will you go through to be released?

_____

_____

_____

List the names of the people you became familiar with on your visit:

(Remember these people when sending thank you notes.)

PREPARING FOR YOUR NEW FAMILY

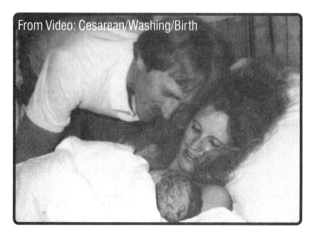

From Video: Cesarean/Washing/Birth

Circumcision: surgically removing the foreskin from a male baby's penis. Done for religious or personal reasons.
Fontanel: normal soft spots or gaps in the skull of the baby.
Hypothermia: abnormally low body temperature.
Incubator: Enclosed, heated, controlled holder for babies.
Jaundice: hyperbilirubinemia; a yellowing of the skin or whites of the eyes.
Meconium: feces of the baby until about the third day.
Molding: the shaping of the baby's head to the shape and size of the birth canal.
Neonatal: pertaining to a newborn baby.
PKU: phenylketonuria; either a test or the name of a disease (inborn error of metabolism) where baby is unable to digest phenylalanine. Can lead to retardation. Very rare (approximately one in 17,000).
Vernix caseosa: "baby cold cream"; white cheesy substance which protects baby's skin in uterus.

Going through the pregnancy, labor and birth is the way we evolve into a new family. This is a new stage of life. It is wonderful in its own way, but it is different and challenging. Remember, millions of families have started out just like yours and have learned to flow with the changes. Take this time to learn, listen and experience. Reduce unnecessary stress and spend as much time together as a family as you can. This time with your new baby will pass very quickly. Babies grow very fast.

In this section, we assume you have had a normal labor and birth and that your baby is healthy and normal. Your Bradley® teacher will be able to refer you to special resources if you have special needs.

SITUATION PRACTICE

This assignment will help to pull together all that you've learned up to this point. By this time, you should be experts at achieving deep relaxation. Remember all that you've learned. Use whichever techniques you feel apply, and practice at least 3 "mock" contractions three minutes apart in the following locations: in your kitchen, in your living room, in your bedroom, in your bathroom, on the toilet, in the bathtub, in the shower, in front of your home, in your car (while coach is driving), in the parking lot at the birth center or hospital (even if you are planning a home birth), in the waiting room, at the market, at the park, and in a restaurant. Are you able to relax in any situation? Can you figure out which techniques work best in each situation? Do you need more practice on anything? You know what you need. Listen to yourself. Continue daily relaxation practice until labor begins. Have a Very Happy Birth-Day!

GENERAL ASSIGNMENTS:

❏ Relaxation: every day.

❏ Walk 30 min 2X a day. Exercises!

❏ Great nutrition: every day... Very Important!

❏ Have good communications with your birth team.

❏ Get plenty of rest.

❏ Keep coming to class till your baby comes.

❏ Read *Student Workbook*, pages 109-112.

❏ Fill out *Student Workbook*, pages 114-115.

❏ Student Center: www.bradleybirth.com

©2010 AAHCC

YOUR NEW BABY

"Babies need love to survive. Social attention is life itself to the human baby." Karen Pryor

Stay in touch with your doctor and La Leche League leader. The following may be helpful.

COLOR

Newborns have a pinky-purple hue from extra blood at birth. This extra blood will be disposed of gradually, which usually gives the baby a yellowish or jaundiced color about the third day after birth. In almost all cases, this is perfectly normal and may even be desirable. Its skin may be covered at birth with a white, cheesy coating called vernix caseosa. Newborns are often born with tiny pearl-like beads (pimples) on the nose and cheeks called milia. These are normal and disappear in a few weeks. Do not try to squeeze them.

APPEARANCE

At birth, your baby will be wet from the amniotic fluid that comes along with birth. The baby may also be bloody, if you had an episiotomy or tear.

HAIR

Babies are born with wet hair that looks darker and, perhaps, curlier when it dries. The color may change completely, later.

STATISTICS

The average baby is 18-22 inches long and weighs 7 1/2 - 9 1/2 pounds.

EYES

In the uterus, babies can distinguish between light and dark. At birth, most babies can see and can follow movement, the ideal focus being the distance from the breastfeeding position to the mother's face. Their eye color often appears dark blue, but it may change days, weeks, or months later. Small blood vessels sometimes burst from the pressure of birth; this is considered normal, and the red streaks go away with time.

CORD

At birth, the average cord is 21" long so most babies can reach the mother's breast before the cord is cut. When it is time, the cord will be clamped with a white plastic clamp, or it can be tied and then cut. In either case, leave these things in place and keep the cord dry. The stump will heal and fall off in approximately 7-14 days. Keep diaper below cord. Your pediatrician may have special instructions about the cord.

GENITALS

If you have a boy, the scrotum may be enlarged. This is normal. If you have a girl, there may be a few drops of blood from the vagina. The breasts of either sex may be enlarged and drops of "witches' milk" may be secreted.

BREATHING

Newborns have irregular, light breathing the first few hours after birth. When sleeping, their breathing is very light. If you are concerned, put your hand on the baby's back and you can feel the baby breathing. Breathing should be easy, with no mucous in the nose or throat. Your physician may want you to have a small bulb syringe on hand.

URINATION

Normally, baby will wet diapers often. If your milk has not come in, the wet diapers may not be as frequent. After three days, the baby will probably have 6 to 8 wet cloth diapers a day. This is a good way to gauge if the baby is getting enough breastmilk. Urine should be clear or very pale yellow.

FIRST BOWEL MOVEMENT

This is called meconium and is a black-green, sticky, tarry substance. It gradually changes to the normal, breastfed bowel movement which is yellow-to-green in color, runny-to-pasty in consistency. It may occur every time you change a diaper or less frequently. Both are normal. The nice thing about the breastfed bowel movement is that it does not have a strong, unpleasant odor.

BREASTFEEDING

Many breastfed babies want to nurse every twenty minutes when they are newborns; gradually this interval lengthens to about two hours. Two hours is still more frequent than bottle-feeding because the breastmilk is easily digested. The baby has a sucking reflex and will turn toward the breast if you touch the nipple to the baby's cheek. PLEASE contact the La Leche League for complete information on breastfeeding.

Class 1
Class 2
Class 3
Class 4
Class 5
Class 6
Class 7
Class 8
Class 9
Class 10
Class 11
Class 12

BREASTFEEDING POSITION

Pay special attention the first few times you breastfeed, making sure the baby gets on the breast correctly. Sit up or lie on your side. Put baby's head in the crook of your arm and hand under buttocks. Turn baby so he is belly to belly with mom. Help to form the nipple by placing your other hand under the breast with thumb on top. Tickle the baby's cheek with your nipple and wait until the baby opens his mouth and has his tongue down. Then pull the baby toward you, with the arm surrounding him, so that as much of the nipple as possible goes into his mouth. Remember, newborns nurse often and the best way to avoid sore nipples is to position the baby correctly on your breast every time.

BURPING

Some babies need to be burped. Others, especially if breastfed, may not. It is not necessary to wake up the baby to burp.

TOUCHING

"The skin of a new baby is far more sensitive than that of an adult. It flushes and mottles at every sensation. It is through his kinesthetic awareness, through being touched and moved and handled, and through the things that touch his sensitive mouth that a baby first locates himself and makes contact with reality."
Karen Pryor *Nursing Your Baby, p.81.*

HICCUPS & SNEEZING

These occur frequently. Newborns often do both, and short periods of both are normal.

SPITTING UP

This is also very normal with some breast and most bottle-fed babies. If your infant is repeatedly vomiting (not just spitting up) with every meal, contact your doctor.

EMOTIONS

Your new baby is immature and its needs should be met quickly, or the response will be crying and distrust of the world. Anthropologist, Ashley Montagu has said that the newborn human infant is at the same stage of development at nine months of age, as other animals are at birth. This means your baby needs almost as much care after birth for the first nine months as it did inside the mother.

Read: *Sweet Dreams* by Dr. Paul Fleiss.

CRYING

All babies cry at times. The cry can be very disturbing to a new parent. Pick up the baby. If the cry is a sudden, high-pitched crying, check all possibilities and, in rare cases when this continues, call your doctor.

INTERACTION

Newborn babies can see, follow and focus. They can also learn. If you smile at your baby he may look right at you and smile back. This is how newborns learn. It is not from gas like so many people say. Your baby can see you and can smile - smile back.

HOLDING

New babies like to be held and often times will cry when you put them down. This may be a signal to you that your baby needs extra touching, rocking, walking and loving. Studies have shown that babies that are held a lot have 70% less crying. You cannot spoil a baby (or anyone else) with too much love.

APGAR

Rating of baby at birth. Each category is given two points.
1. Appearance or Color.
2. Pulse or Heart Rate.
3. Grimace or Responsiveness (Reflex).
4. Activity - Muscle tone.
5. Respiration - Breathing.

List everything that will be done to your baby from the time it is born until released from medical care:

The Bradley Method®

Class 1 | Class 2 | Class 3 | Class 4 | Class 5 | Class 6 | Class 7 | Class 8 | Class 9 | Class 10 | Class 11 | Class 12

NEWBORN PROCEDURES

Tips about

PKU: A test done after birth for a group of conditions including phenylketonuria, galactosemia, and congenital hypothryroidism. This test is generally done with blood taken from the baby's heel or hand. In most states, it is required by state law. This test is sometimes inaccurate and may need to be repeated. In most of these cases, continued breastfeeding is important for these babies.

Eye treatment: Administration of eye prophylaxis is most often a state law. Generally erythromycin or tetracycline ointment is used. Babies experience a short time of discomfort and blurred vision. Waiting 1 or 2 hours will allow for some visual family bonding.

Vitamin K: Vitamin K is a blood-clotting factor that may be given orally or by injection. *Shot or oral drops at birth then 1 week after 1 month after*
* necessary for circumcision
* may increase jaundice

Bundling: Dr. Bradley recommends keeping the baby warm by putting the baby skin-to-skin with the mother, then covering the two of them with blankets, rather than wrapping the baby separately with blankets, shielding it from the radiant heat of the mother's body.

Bathing: You may wish to postpone bathing the baby. It often leads to a drop in the baby's body temperature, causing alarm which may lead to placing the baby in an incubator in the nursery.

Circumcision: Surgical removal of the foreskin is done for social or religious reasons; "there is no absolute medical indication for routine circumcision." (*Guidelines For Perinaral Care*, p. 87). Parents should be as well-informed about circumcision as about any surgery or significant choice they would make on their child's behalf.

Evaluation for jaundice

There are basically 3 types of jaundice in newborns. Jaundice is an often normal and possibly desirable rise in the bilirubin level in the blood. This makes the skin and whites of the eyes look yellow. An excessively high bilirubin level along with a lethargic baby is a danger sign. (This is a rare occurrence.)

Note: La Leche League is a great source of information on newborns.

Types of jaundice

1. **Jaundice of early onset**. This occurs immediately and might indicate a serious problem. It should be evaluated immediately.

2. **Normal physiologic jaundice.** This occurs on or about the third day, is normal, and has been reported that more than 50% of healthy babies have it (*Perinatal Press*, Vol. 7 No. 1). The baby's behavior, breastfeeding frequency, as well as bilirubin levels should be considered during evaluation. Bilirubin is now known to be bacteriostatic and an anti-oxidant, and normal jaundice may be beneficial and even desirable. Remember: jaundice is part of the natural process.

3. **Jaundice of late onset**, Sometimes called breastmilk jaundice. This peaks 10 to 15 days after birth (*Guidelines For Perinatal Care, p.* 221), and is caused by a hormone present in only one in 100-200 women. It is generally not necessary to stop breastfeeding.

Treatment for jaundice

Most types need no treatment, specific treatment will depend on the cause and severity of the condition. Treatments go all the way from blood transfusions, to phototherapy lights, to bottles of special "jaundice" water, to formula, to breastfeeding and sunshine. Rarely should breastfeeding be discontinued.

List things that may increase the incidence of jaundice:
drugs
induced labor
birth control pills prior to pregnancy

List what can be done to help reduce jaundice:
- avoid drugs / induction
- decline vitamin k?

What can you do to handle the pediatric visit when baby is checked for jaundice?
- don't dress the baby in yellow

SUGGESTIONS FOR SUCCESSFUL BREASTFEEDING

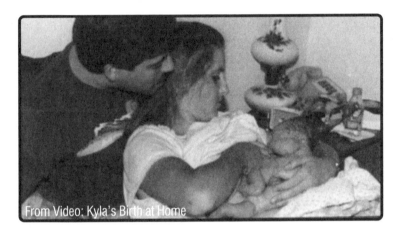

From Video: Kyla's Birth at Home

Dr. E. Robbins Kimball, an advocate of breastfeeding, has helped hundreds of mothers to nurse their babies successfully by sending his patients home with three simple suggestions.

1. Spend your first three days home in bed. Not because you are ill, but because you need plenty of rest, relaxation, and time to develop a relationship with your new baby.

   This means no getting up for anything except to go to the bathroom. Visitors are nice but can be very exhausting for both you and your baby. If you are in bed, it will deter them from overstaying their visit.

   Keep your baby in your bed or in a bed next to it for easy access. If you have another small child at home, simply close your bedroom door and allow him to play in your room. Even 18-month-olds enjoy reading books, drawing, or watching TV with Mother. Have a large bowl of fruit to snack on and a jug of water or juice to drink. This should keep both of you satisfied between meals.

   Forget the housework, laundry, and meals. Allow friends, relatives, and loving husbands to assist you in these areas. Remember, the rest of the household will survive without you for these all-important few days.

2. Take three one-hour naps daily. During the first three days in bed, sleep as often as possible. During the rest of the first month, get into bed and take these three one-hour naps. Sleep: while the children sleep, while your husband plays with the baby, after breakfast, while a neighbor watches the other children. Do not read, watch TV or write, you can do these things while nursing the baby. SLEEP!

   These naps will do more good and do more to make breastfeeding a pleasure with quick success than anything else you do in the first weeks.

3. Remember, it takes two or three weeks to learn how to nurse, and a couple of months to become an expert. Do not regard every little event as a signal for panic. There will be days when you do not have enough milk and days when you have too much. There will be days when your baby appears to go on a "four-hour schedule" and days when he eats all the time. These frequency days are nature's way of increasing your milk supply to keep up with your growing baby's needs. The first two frequency days occur around the fifth and fourteenth days of life.

   You and your baby are both learning; breastfeeding will be easier and easier as you go along.

HAPPY BREASTFEEDING!

Class 1 · Class 2 · Class 3 · Class 4 · Class 5 · Class 6 · Class 7 · Class 8 · Class 9 · Class 10 · Class 11 · Class 12

SOOTHING YOUR BABY

List common reasons babies cry:

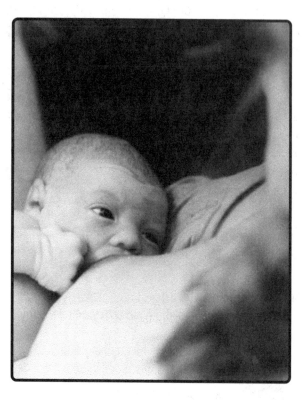

List things you can do to soothe a crying baby:

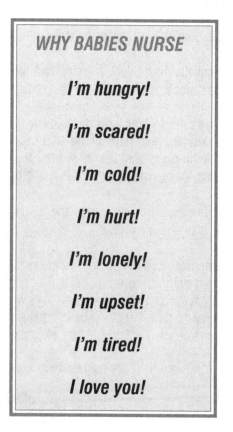

WHY BABIES NURSE

I'm hungry!

I'm scared!

I'm cold!

I'm hurt!

I'm lonely!

I'm upset!

I'm tired!

I love you!

Crying is the baby's means of communication and expression. Most often, you will know what is causing your baby to cry and you'll take care of your baby's needs quickly. You can't now, and won't ever be able to solve all of the pains and problems in your child's life. Do everything you can to soothe your baby, while you comfort and reassure him that you love him no matter what.

Class 1
Class 2
Class 3
Class 4
Class 5
Class 6
Class 7
Class 8
Class 9
Class 10
Class 11
Class 12

MOTHERING

By Susan Hathaway Bek, AAHCC

There may come a time during the last part of your labor, or just before you give the final pushes which will lead to the birth of your baby, when you quietly turn inward and resolve the feelings, doubts, apprehensions and fears you have about becoming a mother.

As a mother who was dedicated to giving my baby a natural childbirth, I found that I had a certain amount of control over my labor. I was able, in a way, to "hold back," as I was unsure of my ability to handle such a big step. At a certain point, I had to sigh. I turned inward, and one last time I reviewed my feelings, I recalled my fears, I remembered my love for my baby and I accepted my responsibility. I held my breath and took that last, big, scary step. Come good or bad, right or wrong, ready or not it was time to begin this adventure. An adventure which would change my life forever.

There will come a time when you, too, must let go of your baby. You will have to stop being pregnant and start being "Mommy."

YOU WILL NOT BE ALONE - You are surrounded by love and support - the loving support of your family, the caring support of your friends. Don't hesitate to call on your Bradley® teacher or La Leche League leader. We know what you're going through. We've been through it too. We want to help.

IT'S GOING TO BE SCARY - Your entire life is about to change. Things will never be the same again and there is no turning back. Life is filled with changes. Very few are as drastic or as scary as this one. Accept the fact that you will be scared. Few paths are as difficult as the one you have chosen, but few offer the opportunity of growth or the abundant pleasure that yours will.

YOU WILL BE AFRAID - Newborn babies seem so fragile and so helpless, and this world we live in seems so harsh. Of course you are going to be afraid. Perhaps it is a good thing that you are. If you were not at times anxious, at times afraid, you would not be as aware of potential dangers - your fear will keep your baby safe.

YOUR INSTINCTS WILL GUIDE YOU - You will be driven to hold and cuddle and touch your baby constantly. You will yearn to hold your baby to your breast and feed him or her. You will be protective and quick to defend your baby. These instincts are vitally important. Don't let anyone deter you from doing that which you know is right.

THE TEARS WILL COME - Be careful not to do too much. Get plenty of rest. You sleep when the baby sleeps! When the tears come, try going for a walk, taking a bath, calling a friend, or just cry with the baby. You'll be learning together, growing together and, yes, crying together. This can make you even closer.

YOU WILL BE COMFORTED - When you put your baby to your breast, and the baby begins to suckle, the warm milk will flow into his body, soothing as well as nourishing him. As this takes place, you will be overcome by a warm, relaxed feeling. You are finally comforted. Remember to nurse your baby often. You will both enjoy the comfort that comes from nursing.

Class 1 | Class 2 | Class 3 | Class 4 | Class 5 | Class 6 | Class 7 | Class 8 | Class 9 | Class 10 | Class 11 | Class 12

RESPONSIBILITY MAY OVERWHELM YOU - Do what you can in advance to lighten your load. Try to get some help with the housework and other responsibilities. Just taking care of yourself and your baby will be all you can handle for awhile. Remember to take one day at a time, one minute at a time if necessary. Take time out to be comforted (you can nurse your baby even if he is not crying for it) and remember that you are not alone.

YOU WILL ADJUST - The first six weeks can be a real challenge. You are changing physically, as well as emotionally. Your baby is changing, too. Give yourselves the time to adjust. After the first six weeks, your nursing will be well-established, you will have physically and emotionally adjusted to no longer being pregnant, you will be more sure of yourself and your mothering abilities, and your baby will have adjusted, too.

YOU'LL MAKE MISTAKES - We all make mistakes- that's part of life. You and your baby will be learning together. Having this in common will make you more understanding.

YOU WILL BE CAPABLE - You will fill your baby's needs as his protector, provider, and healer. Through the fluid which seemingly magically comes from your breasts you will be able to protect your baby from infection and disease, and provide your baby with all of the nourishment that he needs for at least the first six to nine months of his life. A little breastmilk can also help to heal most minor ailments from diaper rash to eye infections.

YOU WILL BE WELL-SUPPLIED - Your milk is produced on a supply and demand basis. Nurse often, and don't give your baby any water, formula or anything except breastmilk and you should always have plenty of milk for your baby.

YOUR CHILD WILL GROW - Pay attention and enjoy this stage of your child's life now. If you're not careful, you might miss it. You will feel a real sense of pride when you look at your child and realize that you are providing all of the nourishment that is causing him or her to grow so fast and so well.

YOUR CONFIDENCE WILL BUILD - With each passing day, you will become more and more confident. You will learn from your mistakes and you will grow from your accomplishments. You will soon realize what a good mother you are!

YOUR JOYS WILL MULTIPLY - Through your child's eyes, you will see the world as few people ever do. You will know the joy of sunshine, the thrill of butterflies, the wonder of a flower and the exhilaration that comes from hearing your child laugh.

YOUR LIFE WILL BE ENRICHED - As you hear your child's first words, as you feel your child's first tooth, as you watch your child's first steps, your life will be enriched.

YOU'LL LEARN, YOU'LL GROW, YOU'LL CHANGE...

YOU'LL NEVER BE THE SAME AGAIN.

The Bradley® Dad:
Eight Keys to an Unbreakable Bond

by Mark A. Moshay, AAHCC

All my life I wanted to be a father. I mean, that was listed as one of my goals. I suppose that one factor has helped me along the way. My three children are very close to their daddy. But I've often thought "Hey, you're not the only one." In fact, most fathers want to be close to their children. Especially today with more time to spend with their families (as opposed to 20 or 30 years ago when dad was but a shadow passing from work shift to work shift), fathers are now more than ever searching for answers to build stronger relationships with their children. Dads everywhere are wondering "just how do I get this bonding thing to work?" Well guys, relax. Hopefully this will help you get a handle on this whole fatherhood experience and you'll be on your way.

To make things a bit more logical, I've divided this topic into eight sub-topics, or "keys." So if you're ready, let's get started.

I. BELLY TALK

It sounds crazy but I did it! I talked to my kids before the dates on their birth certificates. Usually, I would talk to them by putting my mouth up to Jeanne's stomach and say, well, silly things like, "Hey, I can't wait till you come on out." "I know you're going to be a beautiful sweetie." Now I'm not a psychologist (though some have said I should probably see one) nor do I have any hard statistics on the subject, but there are advantages three ways. First, your wife becomes much closer to you because she sees your interest, your concern and most of all, your eagerness to be a part of it all. Second, it gets you more involved because you begin to visualize this soft, warm, little person that you have helped create. Third, (now here comes the crazy part) I actually believe your baby picks up on your tone, voice pattern, and inflections. In other words, you won't be a stranger to him (or her) at the birth scene. After all, it's been pretty well proven that the baby knows mom by smell, touch and sound. I can't prove that this is so with dad, but for all the possible benefits, isn't it worth the few minutes every day or so?

The key here is anticipation and wonder.

II. ADVICE, ADVICE, ADVICE

You'll get a lot. You'll begin to think that everyone from Aunt Sally to the pharmacist is convinced that you're an ignorant moron who couldn't use a toothbrush much less care for a baby. Be patient, smile, and try to bear it. Not easy, but just keep in mind - "I'm going to be the best Dad they ever saw!"

Don't forget all your buddies, "Hey pal, don't let the wife get you changin' diapers," comment. Keep in mind that it's your baby and if you want to change the baby's diaper, you will (I know maybe you don't want to, but I'll get to that later).

On the other hand, don't be afraid to ask questions. The more you ask, the happier your wife will be with your interest. And there is a side benefit, you learn a lot! If anyone gives you any trouble for asking something like "Do babies really bounce?" Just respond like I used to... "Hey that's why I'm asking, I care and I want to do things right."

The key here is to be inquisitive.

III. GO AHEAD-STICK OUT YOUR TONGUE, SON

This is my favorite game to play with newborns, and by golly, it works. I racked my brain in our local library trying to find what kinds of activities a dad can do with a very young child, like let's say three hours old. And there it is! It's as simple as sticking out your tongue. I would look at Shaun and he would watch me as newborns do - kind of entranced. I would stick my tongue out slowly and then hold it out, then back and so on. After about two or three minutes, Jeanne shrieked, "Look honey, he's imitating you." That little guy's tongue was right out there! Jeanne had seen a film that talked about the way even a newborn could react to different stimulus. Sounds real scientific but believe it or not that was one of the "experiments" in the film.

Class 1 · Class 2 · Class 3 · Class 4 · Class 5 · Class 6 · Class 7 · Class 8 · Class 9 · Class 10 · Class 11 · Class 12

The possibilities and variations are endless. Let's see there is blinking, smiling, winking, wrinkling your face, hand waving... Like I said, endless. Be bold and try it-it's fun, it's communication and a reward all it's own.

The key here is contact.

IV. READ TO ME

Jeanne began to read to Shannon, our oldest, when she was only six weeks old. Silly, I thought. But by the time Stephen was born, Shannon was three and a half and starting to read on her own. Coincidence? Well, I tried the same thing with Stephen. Today both children are avid readers and both are in the gifted education program in our local school district. Coincidence?

The key here is early stimulation and interaction

V. YES SIR, THAT'S MY BABY!

I remember vividly and with dread those comments in the park as I strolled with my three year old and infant in my arms. "Oh, stuck with the kids today, huh?" Every time I would have the same answer, "No, I chose to be with them, they are my kids you know."

Hey, you're not alone. You've got a lot of us in your corner. Go for it; be an active dad.

The key here is pride, pride in fatherhood.

VI. LIFE AT GRAND CENTRAL

Yes, you know it will get hectic, plan on it. But, turn it into a plus. Show mom how much you can help her during those frantic times, like ringing phones, water boiling over on the stove and crying babies (all at once, of course). That leads us back to diapers. What? Yes diapers. I changed a lot of them. The wet ones and yes, the other ones too. Hey, don't get me wrong, the idea was not easy for me. But I took it as a challenge. If I can do this, then my wife will know FOR SURE that I care. Nothing is more valuable to me than my photo of Shaun (who was born on my birthday) all sacked out on my chest while I too contentedly checked my eyelids for a positive seal.

The key here is teamwork.

VII. THE PAPA PRINCIPLE

Like the song says, "Nobody does it better." I used to come home at night (I worked swing shift) to Jeanne who would be waiting for me to burp Stephen. Really! I would walk in, give Momma a kiss and grab my little guy. Then, within seconds my mission was complete. I soon learned to grab him with a towel present on my left shoulder. It's something you turn into something special, a memory. Sure, it is kind of gross to a full grown man at first. But stop to think, my wife had been patting him on the back, holding him, and just basically fussing with him for hours. And then like a flash comes Daddy the Wonderman. And as far as what the guys at work might say, well, they don't need to know everything. Again, you will just keep on impressing your wife, yourself, and later on (with new stories to embellish) your child.

The key here is father exclusivity.

And now, the eighth and final key...

VIII. GENETICS, HEREDITY, OR INVOLVEMENT?

Like I said before, two of our three children are in school now and doing well above average... Genetics? Environment? Well, perhaps that is part of it but I'm really convinced that we are witnessing the cycle of involvement that started way back in the 'belly talk' stage. It's two-fold, one is that you were right there all the way with your child (and your wife) and second, your child has grown up in a home of involvement. While the experts battle over genes versus surroundings, it has been our real-life experience that constant involvement is the key and it's contagious! Shaun learned from Stephen. Stephen learned from Shannon. Shannon got her interest in reading from being read to by mom and yes, dad too!

The key is already clear... Involvement, Involvement, Involvement!

In summary, Dad, don't be afraid to be bold and be patient. The rewards are really worth it. Develop your own style and experiment. You will build a stronger marriage and a stronger bond with your children. You'll also find a pride in yourself that no man can match unless he too, has experienced the keys to the unbreakable bond of fatherhood.

Good luck (but you won't really need it - you've got heart and that's the only prerequisite).

TOUCHING MOMENTS

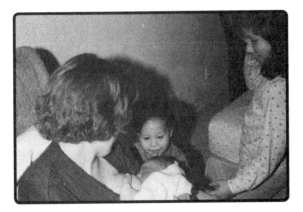
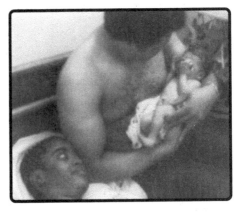
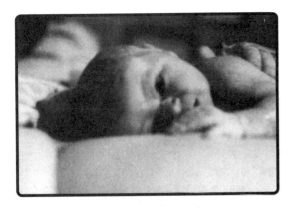
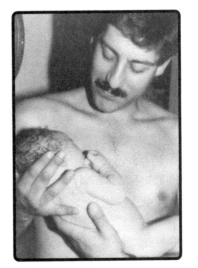
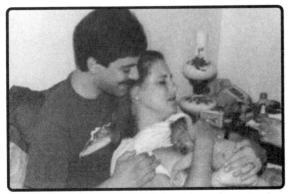
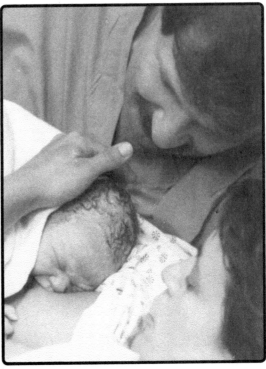
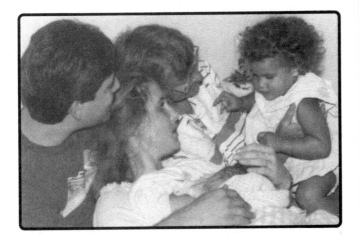

YOUR LABOR AND BIRTH

Family Portrait
(during labor)

This is it! All of the preparation that you have done culminates in these few (or perhaps many) hours of hard work. Remember your training. Use the techniques that you have learned. Concentrate on relaxation. Think about the baby. Stay in touch with your Bradley® teacher. And enjoy taking part in one of the true miracles of life.

Fill in the B.E.S.T. techniques:

A.

B.

C.

D.

E.

F.

G.

H.

I.

J.

K.

L.

M.

N.

O.

P.

Q.

Fill in relaxation and coaching techniques you plan to use in labor:

1.

2.

3.

4.

5.

6.

7.

8.

9.

10.

11.

12.

13.

14.

15.

16.

Class 1
Class 2
Class 3
Class 4
Class 5
Class 6
Class 7
Class 8
Class 9
Class 10
Class 11
Class 12

REFERENCE INFORMATION

Your birth attendant's name:

_____

Phone number: (   )_____

Alternate phone number: (   )_____

Your pediatrician's name:

_____

Phone number: (   )_____

Alternate phone number: (   )_____

Name of your planned birth place:

_____

Phone number: (   )_____

Address:_____

_____

_____

Directions:_____

_____

Draw a map below of how to get from your home to your planned birth place:

In case of emergency, what is the closest hospital that handles obstetrics?

_____

Phone number: (   )_____

Address:_____

_____

Directions:_____

_____

_____

Are there paramedics available in your area? ☐ Yes ☐ No

Phone number: (   )_____

Cost and terms:_____

What is the name of a private ambulance service in your area?

_____

Phone number: (   )_____

Cost and terms:_____

Draw a map below of how to get from your home to the nearest hospital that handles obstetrics:
For emergency use only!

Class 1 Class 2 Class 3 Class 4 Class 5 Class 6 Class 7 Class 8 Class 9 Class 10 Class 11 Class 12

TIMING LATE LABOR CONTRACTIONS

Start	End	Behavior/Comments	Start	End	Behavior/Comments	Start	End	Behavior/Comments

What has changed this hour?

Has she:
  had enough to drink?
  gone to the bathroom?
  been careful to conserve energy?

What techniques have you used?

Mother's comments:

Coach's comments:

What has changed this hour?

Has she:
  had enough to drink?
  gone to the bathroom?
  been careful to conserve energy?

What techniques have you used?

Mother's comments:

Coach's comments:

What has changed this hour?

Has she:
  had enough to drink?
  gone to the bathroom?
  been careful to conserve energy?

What techniques have you used?

Mother's comments:

Coach's comments:

Class 1
Class 2
Class 3
Class 4
Class 5
Class 6
Class 7
Class 8
Class 9
Class 10
Class 11
Class 12

©2010 AAHCC

TIMING LATE LABOR CONTRACTIONS

Start	End	Behavior/Comments		Start	End	Behavior/Comments		Start	End	Behavior/Comments

What has changed this hour?

Has she:
  had enough to drink?
  gone to the bathroom?
  been careful to conserve energy?

What techniques have you used?

Mother's comments:

Coach's comments:

What has changed this hour?

Has she:
  had enough to drink?
  gone to the bathroom?
  been careful to conserve energy?

What techniques have you used?

Mother's comments:

Coach's comments:

What has changed this hour?

Has she:
  had enough to drink?
  gone to the bathroom?
  been careful to conserve energy?

What techniques have you used?

Mother's comments:

Coach's comments:

Class 1 Class 2 Class 3 Class 4 Class 5 Class 6 Class 7 Class 8 Class 9 Class 10 Class 11 **Class 12**

TIMING LATE LABOR CONTRACTIONS

Start	End	Behavior/Comments	Start	End	Behavior/Comments	Start	End	Behavior/Comments

What has changed this hour?

Has she:
  had enough to drink?
  gone to the bathroom?
  been careful to conserve energy?

What techniques have you used?

Mother's comments:

Coach's comments:

What has changed this hour?

Has she:
  had enough to drink?
  gone to the bathroom?
  been careful to conserve energy?

What techniques have you used?

Mother's comments:

Coach's comments:

What has changed this hour?

Has she:
  had enough to drink?
  gone to the bathroom?
  been careful to conserve energy?

What techniques have you used?

Mother's comments:

Coach's comments:

Class 1
Class 2
Class 3
Class 4
Class 5
Class 6
Class 7
Class 8
Class 9
Class 10
Class 11
Class 12

TIMING LATE LABOR CONTRACTIONS

Start	End	Behavior/Comments	Start	End	Behavior/Comments	Start	End	Behavior/Comments

What has changed this hour?

Has she:
  had enough to drink?
  gone to the bathroom?
  been careful to conserve energy?

What techniques have you used?

Mother's comments:

Coach's comments:

What has changed this hour?

Has she:
  had enough to drink?
  gone to the bathroom?
  been careful to conserve energy?

What techniques have you used?

Mother's comments:

Coach's comments:

What has changed this hour?

Has she:
  had enough to drink?
  gone to the bathroom?
  been careful to conserve energy?

What techniques have you used?

Mother's comments:

Coach's comments:

Class 1
Class 2
Class 3
Class 4
Class 5
Class 6
Class 7
Class 8
Class 9
Class 10
Class 11
Class 12

Class 1
Class 2
Class 3
Class 4
Class 5
Class 6
Class 7
Class 8
Class 9
Class 10
Class 11
Class 12

THE STORY OF OUR BIRTH

You will be surprised how quickly you forget important details of your birth. We suggest you write them down as soon as possible. Be sure to include the following: how you prepared, what you expected, how labor began, active first stage, transition, second stage, the birth, what Mommy first said, what Daddy first said, and your first week together.

Class 1
Class 2
Class 3
Class 4
Class 5
Class 6
Class 7
Class 8
Class 9
Class 10
Class 11
Class 12

To Be Continued. . .

THE _____ FAMILY

Family Portrait
(after birth)

Congratulations! We hope that you have many, many fond memories of your birth. We realize that labor and birth are very complex events and expect that you have many differing emotions at this time. We suggest that you pat yourselves on the back for doing your best and savor the good moments. We have enjoyed taking part in this very special time in your lives. We hope that you will keep in touch with your Bradley® teacher and please be sure to complete your follow-up card and send it in to the Academy. We really appreciate your input. Best wishes to you and your wonderful new family!

Baby's Name: _____

Birth Date: _____

Time of Birth: _____ ☐A.M ☐P.M.

Baby's Weight: ____ lbs. ____ oz. *Length:* _____

Hair Color: _____ *Eye Color:* _____

Birth Team: _____ *Comments:* _____

_____ _____

_____ _____

©2010 AAHCC

Class 1
Class 2
Class 3
Class 4
Class 5
Class 6
Class 7
Class 8
Class 9
Class 10
Class 11
Class 12

BREWER PREGNANCY DIET...
A WELL BALANCED PREGNANCY DIET CONSISTS OF:

Every day of the week you and your baby should have:

Milk Products: One quart (4 glasses) or more of milk. Any kind will do: whole milk, low fat, skim, buttermilk, or cheese, yogurt, ice cream, etc....
(Provides protein, calcium, and other essential vitamins & minerals.)

Eggs: Two eggs, (hard boiled, in french toast, or added to other foods).
(Provides protein, vitamins & minerals, including vitamin A and necessary cholesterol.)

Protein: Two servings of fish or seafood, liver, chicken, lean beef, lamb or pork, beans or any kind of cheese.
(Provides amino acids which are the building blocks of the body.)

Greens: Two good servings of fresh green leafy vegetables: mustard, collard, turnip greens, spinach, lettuce, or cabbage.
(Provides minerals and folic acid, also rich in vitamins.)

Whole grains: Four or more slices of whole grain wheat bread, corn bread, cereal, or tortillas.
(Provides carbohydrates for fuel and B vitamins necessary for growth of nerve tissues.)

Vitamin C Foods: One or two pieces of citrus fruit or glass of juice of lemon, lime, orange, tomato, or grapefruit.
(Important in your body's defense system, iron absorption and tissue strength.)

Butter (Fats & Oils): Three servings of butter, or flax seed oil, avocados, olive oil, etc..
(Needed to help absorb fat-soluble vitamins, skin stretchability and energy.)

Fruits & Vegetables: One serving each day of other fruits and vegetables.
(Provide fiber, vitamins, and minerals needed for growth.)

Also include in your diet:

1. A yellow or orange-colored fruit or vegetable five times a week.
   (Provides vitamin A which helps to prevent infections.)
2. Liver once a week. (if you like it)
   (Good source of: protein, vitamins & minerals.)
3. Whole baked potato three times a week.
   (Good source of nutrients.)
4. Plenty of fluids, water, juice etc..
   (Prevents dehydration.)
5. Salt food to taste for a safe increase in blood volume.
   (Helps to maintain equilibrium of body fluids... Essential!)

You may substitute proteins if you wish, being sure your proteins are complete, and that you get approximately 80-100 grams per day. If you substitute, also be sure all the elements necessary for a well balanced diet are available every day. If you substitute for milk, be sure you include protein, calcium and calories in your calculations.

Dr. Thomas Brewer is the foremost authority on nutrition in pregnancy today. Dr. Brewer has been instrumental in the evolution of having healthy mothers, babies and pregnancies. Without his dedication... malnourished mothers might still be the norm!!! Thank you Dr. Brewer.

PROTEIN COUNTER

Dairy Products
Milk, (1C)......................8gm
Cheddar/Swiss, (1oz)......7gm
Processed Cheese,(1oz).6gm
Cottage Cheese, (1/2C) ..12gm
Ice Cream, (1C)................6gm
Yogurt, (1C)....................7gm
Butter, (1tbsp)..............0.1gm
Sour cream, (1oz).......2.25gm
Cream cheese, (1oz)....2gm

Meats
Bologna, (1oz)..............3.8gm
Beef, (3oz)......................20gm
Chicken, (3oz)................25gm
Egg, (1).............................6gm
Hot Dog, (1)......................7gm
Turkey, (3oz)..................27gm
Pork, (3oz)......................21gm
Liver, (3.5oz)..............26gm
Sausage, links (4oz.).......11gm

Fish
Crabmeat, cooked (4oz)..14gm
Clams, steamed (4oz)..12gm
Haddock, (3oz)........16gm
Salmon, (3oz)..............17gm
Shrimp, (4oz)..............20gm
Halibut, (3.5oz)..........26gm
Tuna, canned (4oz)........28gm
Scallops, baked (4oz)....17gm
Lobster, steamed (4oz)..19gm

Carbohydrates
Potato, (medium)............2gm
Rice, Brown (1C)..............6gm
Corn, (1C)........................5gm
Egg Plant, cooked (1C)......2gm
Squash, cooked (1C)........2gm
Kale, cooked (1C)............5gm
Noodles, (1C)..................6gm

Sweet Potato, (medium).......2gm
Bread, (1slice)..................2gm
Crackers, (4Saltines)...........1gm
Doritos, (9/16oz)...............1gm
Fritos, (1oz).....................2gm
Potato Chips, (16pcs).....0.8gm
Tortillas, (1).....................1.2gm

Cereals
Cheerios, (1.25C)...........3.8gm
Granola, (1/4C)...................4gm
Shredded Wheat, (2/3C)........3gm
Wheat Germ, (1tbsp)...........2gm

Nuts
Peanut Butter, (1tbsp).........4gm
Peanuts, (1/4C)...................9gm
Walnuts, (1/4C)...................6gm
Sesame seeds (2oz)...........5gm
Sunflower seeds-hlled(2oz)13gm
Almonds, (4oz)...................21gm
Cashews, (4oz)..................19gm
Pecans, (4oz)...................10gm

Beans
Pinto Beans, (1/2C)..............7gm
Navy Beans, (1/2C)..............7gm
Kidney Beans, (1/2C)...........7gm
Soybean curd-Tofu, (4oz)....9gm
Soy sauce, (1tbsp).............1gm
Soymilk pwdr-dry (1oz)......12gm

Fruit & Juice
Avocado, (large).................4gm
Apple, (medium)..............0.3gm
Cranberry juice, (1C)...........trace
Grapefruit juice, (1C)............1gm
Grapes, (1C).....................1gm
Lemon, (medium)............2.5gm
Nectarine, (medium)...........1gm
Orange, (medium).............1.6gm

Peach, (medium)..............0.6gm
Pineapple juice, (1C)............1gm
Pumpkin, raw (1C)..............2.5gm
Strawberry, (1C)..................1gm
Watermelon, (1slice)...........2gm
Cantaloupe, (1/4)................1gm
Tomato juice, (1C)...............2gm
Vegetable Juice, (4oz)........1gm
Grape Juice, (4oz)............0.3gm
Orange Juice, (1/2C)............1gm
Tangerine, (1med)..............1gm
Raisin, (1/2C)......................2gm
Raspberry, (1C)................0.5gm
Rhubarb, cooked (1C)..........1gm

Vegetables
Asparagus, (6spears)..........2gm
Broccoli, (1C)......................5gm
Carrot, (1)........................0.6gm
Celery, (1lg.stalk)..............0.3gm
Lettuce, (1/2C)..................0.3gm
Cucumber, (1/8lbs)...........0.2gm
Tomato, (1)........................1gm
Spinach, raw (1/4C)............1gm
Cabbage, cooked (1/2C)....1.2gm
Green Beans, (1/2C)..........0.8gm
Cauliflower, cooked (1C).......3gm
Beets, cooked (1C)..............2gm
Onions, (1C)....................2.5gm
Eggplant, (1C)....................2gm

Soups
Vegetable Soup, (1C)............3gm
Beef Broth, (1C)..................5gm
Chicken Noodle, (1C)...........8gm

Sugar Foods
Colas, ...0gm
White Sugar, ...0gm
Caramels,..........................trace
Honey, (2Tbsp)....................trace

Resource infomation for this worksheet: *Nutrition during Pregnancy and Lactation* from California Department of Health, *Husband-Coached Childbirth* by Robert Bradley, M.D., *Nourishing Your Unborn Child* by Phyllis Williams, *What Every Pregnant Woman Should Know* by Gail Brewer, *Introductory Nutrition* by Helen Guthrie, and *Composition of Foods* United States Department of Agriculture.

FIRST STAGE POSITIONS

©2010 AAHCC

NOTES

CERTIFICATE OF CONGRATULATIONS

_____ AND _____

Prepared Mother   Trained labor and birth coach

Are graduates of
The Bradley Method®
Having attended classes, lectures, videos,
and studied the natural process of birth.

Be it known to all who witness this certificate
that this child,

_____

Baby's name

born on: _____

was brought into this world
knowingly with great joy!

This Certificate Acknowledges the
Title of
"PARENTS"

American Academy®
of
Husband-Coached
Childbirth

_____

Bradley® Instructor